PREP

PROGRAM REVIEW & EXAM PREPARATION

ESSENTIALS OF
ACLS

PREP

PROGRAM REVIEW & EXAM PREPARATION

ESSENTIALS OF ACLS

C. A. Brainard, BA, RRT, RCP
Associate Professor
Health and Emergency Services Department
Crafton Hills College
Yucaipa, California

With Contributions by
Ross Nye Giem, BA, MD, FACS, ACEP
Emergency Medicine, General Surgery
Urgent Care Centers, Inc.
Long Beach, California

Medical Illustrations and ECG strips by
Rick R. Schneblin, TGA, BG

APPLETON & LANGE
Stamford, Connecticut

97 98 99 00 01 / 10 9 8 7 6 5 4 3 2 1

Prentice Hall International (UK) Limited, *London*
Prentice Hall of Australia Pty. Limited, *Sydney*
Prentice Hall Canada, Inc., *Toronto*
Prentice Hall Hispanoamericana, S.A., *Mexico*
Prentice Hall of India Private Limited, *New Delhi*
Prentice Hall of Japan, Inc., *Tokyo*
Simon and Schuster Asia Pte. Ltd., *Singapore*
Editora Prentice Hall do Brasil Ltda., *Rio de Janeiro*
Prentice Hall, *Upper Saddle River, New Jersey*

Library of Congress Cataloging-in-Publication Data

Brainard, C. A., 1947–
    Essentials of ACLS : program review and exam preparation / C.A.
  Brainard; with contributions by Ross Nye Giem; medical
  illustrations and ECG strips by Rick R. Schneblin.
        p.   cm.
    Includes index.
    ISBN 0-8385-0259-8 (pbk. : alk. paper)
    1. Cardiovascular emergencies—Treatment—Outlines, syllabi, etc.
  2. CPR (First aid)—Outlines, syllabi, etc.   3. Cardiac arrest—
  Treatment—Outlines, syllabi, etc.   4. Arrhythmia—Treatment—
  Outlines, syllabi, etc.   I. Giem, Ross Nye.   II. Title.
    [DNLM: 1. Cardiopulmonary Resuscitation—methods.   2. First Aid—
  methods.   WA 292 B814e 1997]
  RC675.B73   1997
  616.1'025—dc21
  DNLM/DLC
  for Library of Congress   96-48081
                                                              CIP

Acquisitions Editor: Marinita Timban
Production Editor: Elizabeth Ryan
Designer: Libby Schmitz
Production Service: Rainbow Graphics, Inc.

PRINTED IN THE UNITED STATES OF AMERICA

ISBN 0-8385-0259-8   NB2I

9 780838 502594   90000

Dedication

To my parents: *For their support*
To Susan & Kevin: *For their love*
To Ross: *For his knowledge*
To our students: *For inspiring us*

Contents

Preface

As health professionals, the driving force behind our work is the desire to provide ever better care. Unfortunately these efforts often collide with fiscal restraints.

As the force of managed care is applied and as regulatory agencies escalate reporting requirements, practitioners find themselves pulled in a number of directions. Administrators respond by asking us to broaden our base of knowledge and skills. As the number of services provided multiplies, so do our educational needs.

As we move into the twenty-first century, continuing education becomes increasingly important. To this end, providers on every tier find help in the educational programs offered by the American Heart Association.

Improving our basic and advanced life support skills, and supporting efforts to increase the number of individuals who provide them, leaves no community of interest unserved. Overwhelming evidence exists that the most fractional decrements in rescuer response time yield significant increases in survival rates. Thus, improvements in the delivery of CPR and emergency cardiac care constitutes one of the surest ways to enhance patient outcomes and cost containment efforts.

It is our hope that reviewing this material will not only assist your ACLS educational process, but reinforce the love of learning so vital to our professional growth and development.

INTENDED AUDIENCE

This text is specifically designed for pre-hospital and acute/sub-acute facility health care providers preparing for an "Essentials of ACLS" course.

An *Essentials of ACLS* course provides coverage of the nine essential ACLS case scenarios and the algorithms they are constructed around. These cases and their respective algorithms are listed below. For a detailed discussion of "Essential" and "Comprehensive" ACLS courses and their curricula please refer to Chapter 1: ACLS Course Requirements:

- Case I: Respiratory Arrest With a Pulse/The Universal Algorithm
- Case II: Witnessed Cardiac Arrest/The AED Algorithm
- Case III: Refractory VF/VT/The VF/VT Algorithm
- Case IV: Pulseless Electrical Activity/The PEA Algorithm
- Case V: Asystole/The Asystole Algorithm

- Case VI: Acute Myocardial Infarction/The Acute Myocardial Infarction Algorithm
- Case VII: Unstable Bradycardia/The Bradycardia Algorithm
- Case VIII: Unstable Tachycardia/The Electrical Cardioversion Algorithm
- Case IX: Stable Tachycardia/The Stable Tachycardia Algorithm

OUTSTANDING FEATURES

This text reviews the most recent *guidelines* and *recommendations* for providing adult ACLS. Its purpose is to help health care professionals become ACLS providers. It is designed to prepare course participants for the problem-oriented, *case-based ACLS educational process.*

As such, it is built on and gives frequent attribution to the guidelines and recommendations brought forth in the following publications:

1. American Heart Association. Guidelines for cardiopulmonary resuscitation and emergency cardiac care. JAMA 1992;268:2171–2302.
2. American Heart Association. Textbook for Advanced Cardiac Life Support. Dallas: American Heart Association, 1994.
3. American Heart Association. Instructors Manual for Advanced Cardiac Life Support. Dallas: American Heart Association, 1994.

An important feature of this text is that its content is limited to the knowledge and skills designated by the AHA's Instructor's Manual for ACLS as being part of an *Essential ACLS Provider* course (see Chapter 1). As a result, participants can better allocate study time to strengthen areas of weakness.

This book also provides a comprehensive but concise review of arrhythmia recognition and pharmacology. Again, only those arrhythmias and therapeutic agents designated as "essential" or "core" are reviewed.

Most importantly, this text devotes an entire chapter to the critical actions that must be performed in each of the ACLS case management stations. To obtain providership, participants must *demonstrate proficiency* by successfully managing each of the nine case scenarios listed above. Chapter 13, The Essential ACLS Cases, specifically details performance skills which must be demonstrated as well as the unacceptable errors for each case.

Finally, to help course participants prepare for the ACLS written examination, this text features a sample ACLS written exam meant to be taken as a course pretest. It also features another ACLS written exam that should be taken as a post-test.

WHAT THIS BOOK IS NOT

Used by the authors over the last twenty years, this text represents a successful approach to strengthening core ACLS related knowledge and skills. It is drawn from and throughout properly gives attribution to the JAMA 1992;268:2171-2302: Guidelines for CPR and Emergency Cardiac Care.

A review book such as this is *not* a substitute for standard textbooks and reference works in a field of endeavour. Accordingly ACLS course participants should also obtain the AHA Textbook of Advanced Cardiac Life Support.

These references are comprehensive and definitive sources of information regarding ACLS. The study of advanced cardiac life support must thus be built on the solid foundation they provide. For the individual possessing this reservoir of knowledge, a review text such as this will be a valuable asset indeed.

Acknowledgments

Thanks are in order for the editorial staff at Appleton & Lange for their encouragement and patience. This project could not have advanced without the support of Marinita Timban, Review Book Editor, and Amy Schermerhorn, Editorial Associate.

I would also like to take this time to thank Rick and Julie Schneblin for their manuscript preparation efforts.

Comments and criticisms regarding this text are encouraged and should be directed to Appleton & Lange.

C. A. Brainard, BA, RRT, RCP

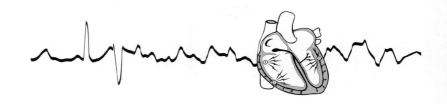

ESSENTIALS OF ACLS PRETEST

1. Which of the following arrhythmias is responsible for the majority of episodes of adult nontraumatic cardiac arrest?
   a. asystole
   b. third-degree atrioventricular (AV) block
   c. idioventricular rhythms
   d. ventricular fibrillation

2. An electrocardiographic indication for considering thrombolytic therapy would be the presence of ST segment elevation of at least 1 mm in two contiguous leads on a 12-lead ECG.
   a. true
   b. false

3. Useful drugs in the treatment of cardiogenic shock include
   1. norepinephrine
   2. nitroprusside
   3. diltiazem
   4. dopamine
   a. 2, 4
   b. 1, 4
   c. 1, 2, 3
   d. 1, 2, 4

4. A patient presents to the emergency department with chest pain and light-headedness. The blood pressure is 75/40 mm Hg. The monitor shows a second-degree type II AV block with wide ventricular complexes occurring at a rate of 35/min. The *initial* therapeutic modality is?
   a. transcutaneous pacing (TCP)
   b. atropine
   c. isoproterenol
   d. dopamine

5. Endotracheal intubation
    1. is indicated in alert and conscious individuals
    2. may result in esophageal intubation
    3. assists management of acidosis during cardiac arrest
    4. helps protect the airway from aspiration of gastric contents
    a. 1, 3, 4
    b. 2, 3, 4
    c. 1, 2, 4
    d. all of the above

6. Bag–valve–mask devices
    1. may require two rescuers for effective use
    2. can be used by untrained individuals
    3. always deliver larger tidal volumes than mouth-to-mask ventilation
    4. can provide oxygen concentrations that approach 100%
    a. 1, 4
    b. 2, 4
    c. 1, 3, 4
    d. all of the above

7. Acidosis that results during cardiac arrest
    1. may be worsened by the administration of sodium bicarbonate
    2. should be managed initially by intubation, ventilation, and car-
       diopulmonary resuscitation (CPR)
    3. is best prevented by restoration of a perfusing rhythm
    4. cannot be treated by administering sodium bicarbonate
    a. 1, 2, 4
    b. 1, 2, 3
    c. 2, 3, 4
    d. all of the above

8. Suctioning through an endotracheal (ET) tube
    1. should be preceded by hyperoxygenation
    2. should not exceed 5 seconds
    3. can result in arrhythmias
    4. can be performed using rigid pharyngeal tip devices
    a. 1, 2, 4
    b. 1, 3, 4
    c. 2, 3
    d. 1, 3

9. Ventilation via an endotracheal tube
    1. should utilize tidal volumes that are 10 to 15 mL/kg
    2. can be performed asynchronously with CPR
    3. should utilize 100% oxygen
    4. is a mainstay in managing acidosis during cardiac arrest

a. 2, 3, 4
b. 1, 3, 4
c. 1, 2, 3
d. all of the above

10. To assure proper endotracheal tube placement, the first place one should auscultate is
    a. over both lung apices anteriorly
    b. over both lung bases anteriorly
    c. over both lung bases posteriorly
    d. over the epigastrium

11. A malleable stylet is used during endotracheal intubation to
    a. reduce the risk of aspiration
    b. help visualize the vocal cords
    c. help the tube conform to the structure of the upper airways
    d. eliminates the need for cricoid pressure

12. Cricoid pressure during endotracheal intubation
    1. should be maintained until the tube cuff is inflated
    2. help prevent gastric aspiration
    3. is not necessary during cardiac arrest
    4. does not require a second rescuer
    a. 1, 2
    b. 2, 4
    c. 1, 3, 4
    d. 1, 2, 4

13. Transcutaneous pacing
    1. presents the hazard of operator shock
    2. may result in patient discomfort
    3. may be used as a bridge mechanism for complete heart block
    4. is a class I intervention for all symptomatic bradycardias
    a. 1, 3, 4
    b. 2, 3, 4
    c. 1, 2, 3
    d. all of the above

14. The *initial* energy recommendation for electrical conversion of paroxysmal supraventricular tachycardia (PSVT) is
    a. 25 J
    b. 50 J
    c. 100 J
    d. 200 J

15. Transthoracic impedance is known to decrease with
    1. greater paddle pressure
    2. larger paddle size

3. successive countershocks
4. use of conductive media
   a. 1, 3, 4
   b. 2, 3, 4
   c. 1, 2, 4
   d. all of the above

16. A dobutamine infusion greater than 20 μg/kg/min will likely result in
    a. unwanted tachycardia
    b. mesenteric arterial dilitation
    c. decreased myocardial contractility
    d. pronounced systemic arterial hypertension

17. In the treatment of stable wide-complex tachycardias of uncertain origin, the following are indicated. Which is the correct intervention sequence?
    1. adenosine
    2. procainamide
    3. lidocaine
    4. bretylium
    a. 3, 4, 2, 1
    b. 3, 2, 4, 1
    c. 3, 1, 2, 4
    d. 3, 1, 4, 2

18. Which of the following interventions is *least* advisable in treating symptomatic bradycardias?
    a. isoproterenol
    b. dopamine
    c. transcutaneous pacing
    d. atropine

19. Which of the following drugs is *least* likely to result in successful treatment of stable ventricular tachycardia (VT)?
    a. lidocaine
    b. bretylium
    c. verapamil
    d. procainamide

20. Patients with acute substernal chest pain radiating to the left arm who present to the emergency department
    1. often deny symptom severity
    2. should receive nitroglycerin and morphine
    3. should receive furosemide
    4. should receive oxygen, IV access, and monitoring
    a. 1, 2, 4
    b. 2, 3, 4

c. 1, 2, 3
d. all of the above

21. A patient with pulseless electrical activity (PEA) is seen in the emergency department. CPR is being performed, the patient is intubated, and IV access has just been obtained. The next intervention should be
a. epinephrine 1 mg
b. atropine 0.5 to 1.0 mg
c. an echocardiogram
d. calcium chloride 5 mL of a 10% solution

22. Failure to recognize and treat third-degree AV block is most likely to lead to
a. ventricular fibrillation
b. asystole
c. atrial fibrillation
d. Torsade de pointes

23. During cardiac arrest, central veins
1. are preferred only if catheterized prior to arrest
2. are associated with hazards such as tension pneumothorax and hematoma
3. allow drugs to reach central organs most rapidly
4. are preferred because interruptions to CPR are minimal
a. 1, 2, 3
b. 1, 2, 4
c. 2, 3
d. all of the above

24. If sodium bicarbonate is indicated in an adult cardiac arrest patient, the patient should receive
a. one ampule (50 mEq), and then one-half of the initial dose every ten minutes
b. 1 mEq/kg initially and one-half the initial dose every ten minutes
c. 50 mEq every ten minutes
d. 100 mEq every ten minutes

25. Six minutes after a witnessed cardiac arrest, quick-look paddles reveal a fine ventricular fibrillation. Which of the following would you recommend?
a. resume CPR, intubate, administer epinephrine, and defibrillate times three
b. resume CPR, charge defibrillator to 360 joules, and defibrillate times three using full power
c. resume CPR, give lidocaine, charge the defibrillator, and defibrillate times three using 200 J, 220 to 300 J, and 360 J
d. resume CPR, charge defibrillator, and defibrillate times three using 200 J, 200 to 300 J, and 360 J

26. Which of the following is *least* likely to be included in the initial treatment of the patient with suspected myocardial infarction?
    a. an IV line
    b. 12-lead ECG
    c. norepinephrine
    d. morphine

27. Present evidence indicates that the dose of drugs injected into the adult tracheobronchial tree should be
    a. 1.0 to 1.5 times the recommended IV dose in 10 mL of solution
    b. 2.0 to 2.5 times the recommended IV dose in 20 mL of solution
    c. 3.0 to 3.5 times the recommended IV dose in 20 mL of solution
    d. 2.0 to 2.5 times the recommended IV dose in 10 mL of solution

28. Atropine
    1. has a dosage end point of 0.04 mg/kg
    2. is indicated for symptomatic bradycardias
    3. may increase myocardial oxygen demands
    4. must be used with caution in patients with acute myocardial infarction (AMI)
    a. 1, 2, 4
    b. 2, 3, 4
    c. 1, 3, 4
    d. all of the above

29. Nitroglycerin
    1. may be given as a paste or a spray
    2. can only cause hypotension when given IV
    3. is often preferred over nitroprusside in the ACLS setting
    4. is associated with increases in infarct size
    a. 2, 3
    b. 1, 4
    c. 2, 4
    d. 1, 3

30. Sodium bicarbonate
    1. is believed to be useful in cardiac arrest involving pre-existing acidosis
    2. should not be used to treat hypoxic lactic acidosis
    3. may be useful in prolonged cardiac arrest if the patient is intubated
    4. is believed to be useful in cardiac arrest involving pre-existing hyperkalemia
    a. 1, 3, 4
    b. 2, 3, 4
    c. 1, 2, 3
    d. all of the above

31. All of the following are indicated in the treatment of ventricular fibril-
    lation (VF). Please place them in their proper sequence.
    1. epinephrine 1 mg IV push
    2. three initial attempts at defibrillation
    3. endotracheal intubation/IV access
    4. defibrillation at 360 J
    a. 2, 1, 3, 4
    b. 2, 3, 1, 4
    c. 2, 3, 4, 1
    d. 2, 1, 4, 3

32. The correct energy sequence for the three initial attempts at adult de-
    fibrillation is
    a. 200 J, 200 to 300 J, 400 J
    b. 200 J, 300 J, 360 J
    c. 200 J, 200 to 300 J, 360 J
    d. 100 J, 300 J, 360 J

33. Your first action on discovering a patient who is in asystole is
    to
    a. defibrillate at 200 J
    b. administer epinephrine
    c. provide IV access
    d. confirm its presence in more than one lead

34. A patient is seen in the emergency department. He has crushing chest
    pain and altered consciousness. His BP is 70/50 mm Hg. The monitor
    reveals a rapid ventricular tachycardia. Select the correct intervention
    sequence.
    a. cardiovert using 100 J, 200 J, 300 J, 360 J
    b. lidocaine, procainamide, bretylium
    c. lidocaine, bretylium, procainamide
    d. lidocaine, adenosine, procainamide

35. A narrow-complex stable PSVT that does not respond to vagal ma-
    neuvers and two doses of adenosine should be treated next with
    a. synchronized cardioversion
    b. verapamil 2.5 to 5 mg IV
    c. verapamil 5 to 10 mg IV
    d. beta blockers

36. A 55-year-old, 75-kg female is brought to the emergency department
    via the EMS system. She is complaining of crushing chest pain. The
    BP is 160/100 mm Hg. The monitor shows sinus tachycardia with fre-
    quent premature ventricular contractions (PVCs). You would recom-
    mend
    1. oxygen
    2. 12-lead ECG

3. nitroglycerin and morphine
4. lidocaine
a. 1, 2, 3
b. 2, 3, 4
c. 1, 2
d. all of the above

37. A 50-kg patient is brought to the emergency department after having suffered syncope. His BP is 82/50 mm Hg, and the cardiac monitor shows a second-degree type II rhythm with block at the infranodal level. The ventricular rate is 38/min. Select the *definitive* intervention for this patient.
    a. atropine 0.5 to 1 mg IV push
    b. transvenous pacing
    c. dopamine 5 to 20 μg/kg/min
    d. transcutaneous pacing

38. While performing cardioversion, the patient becomes pulseless. Select the correct next intervention.
    a. cardioversion
    b. CPR
    c. defibrillation
    d. epinephrine

39. Which of the following forms of therapy would you employ initially for a pulseless patient with VF?
    a. synchronized countershock
    b. epinephrine
    c. volume infusion
    d. CPR

40. A severely distressed patient is brought to the emergency department complaining of chest pain, palpitations, and shortness of breath. The BP is 75/50, and the monitor reveals a wide complex tachycardia with a rate of 220/min. You would recommend
    a. verapamil 5 mg IV
    b. lidocaine 1 mg/kg IV
    c. synchronized cardioversion at 200 J
    d. synchronized cardioversion at 50 J to 100 J

41. Which of the following are part of the differential diagnostic process to be employed in searching for treatable causes of PEA?
    1. a volume infusion
    2. examination of neck veins
    3. auscultation of the lungs
    4. assessment of blood flow
    a. 1, 2, 3
    b. 2, 3, 4

c. 1, 3, 4
d. all of the above

42. In the context of possible acute myocardial infarction (AMI), which of the following are routinely employed?
 1. morphine
 2. volume infusion
 3. lidocaine
 4. oxygen
 a. 1, 3,
 b. 2, 3
 c. 2, 4
 d. 1, 4

43. All of the following IV drugs may be indicated in the treatment of symptomatic bradycardias. Please place them in their proper sequence.
 1. dopamine infusion
 2. epinephrine infusion
 3. isoproterenol infusion
 4. atropine IV bolus
 a. 4, 2, 1, 3
 b. 4, 2, 3, 1
 c. 4, 1, 3, 2
 d. 4, 1, 2, 3

44. *Absolute* contraindications to thrombolytic therapy include
 1. recent stroke
 2. active internal bleeding
 3. symptom duration greater than 6 hours
 4. age greater than 70 years
 a. 1, 2, 4
 b. 1, 2,
 c. 1, 2, 3
 d. 1, 3, 4

45. Signs that PEA may be due to cardiac tamponade include
 1. jugular venous distention
 2. weak or absent pulse during CPR
 3. improvement in response to fluid challenge
 4. history of chest trauma, recent CPR
 a. 1, 2, 4
 b. 1, 2, 3
 c. 2, 3
 d. all of the above

46. Which of the following therapeutic agents *cannot* be administered via an endotracheal tube?
    a. atropine
    b. naloxone
    c. lidocaine
    d. sodium bicarbonate

47. When establishing IV access during cardiac arrest, it is important to remember that
    1. veins in the antecubital fossa do not require interruption of CPR
    2. some agents can be given endotracheally
    3. strict aseptic technique is mandatory
    4. catheters be as large as is practicable
    a. 1, 3, 4
    b. 2, 3, 4
    c. 1, 2, 3,
    d. 1, 2, 4

48. Stable atrial flutter with a rapid ventricular response, would best be treated with which of the following modalities?
    a. dobutamine
    b. diltiazem
    c. atropine
    d. lidocaine

49. A patient is seen in the emergency department following an AMI. The patient has complaints of shortness of breath and chest pain. His BP is 150/90 mm Hg. His respiratory rate is 25/min, and bilateral rales can be heard on auscultation. The monitor shows sinus tachycardia with frequent PVCs. Useful agents include
    1. furosemide
    2. nitroglycerin IV
    3. dopamine
    4. morphine
    a. 1, 2, 3
    b. 2, 3, 4
    c. 1, 2, 4
    d. 1, 3, 4

50. When the "no shock indicated" command is issued by an automated external defibrillator (AED) device, the rescuer's next intervention is to
    a. activate the analysis control
    b. resume CPR
    c. check for presence of pulse
    d. call for help

ESSENTIALS OF ACLS PRETEST: WRITTEN REFERENCED ANSWERS

The questions presented in the foregoing test were constructed to measure the same knowledge and skills as do the items on the actual ACLS written examination.

To help course participants prepare for the ACLS examination process, each question is discussed and referenced to the following AHA publications.

Reference I:
American Heart Association. Guidelines for CPR and ECC. JAMA 1992;268: 2171–2302

Reference II:
American Heart Association. Textbook for advanced cardiac life support. Dallas, TX: American Heart Association, 1994

Reference III:
American Heart Association. Instructor's manual for ACLS. Dallas, TX: American Heart Association, 1994

Following each discussion, the question will be referenced to one of the three standard texts mentioned above. Following the reference citation (eg, reference I, reference II, etc.) will come the pages(s) or chapter and page number(s) that can be used to obtain additional information.

1. Answer . . . d.

Approximately 80 to 90% of episodes of adult nontraumatic cardiac arrest are due to VF/VT. Accordingly, the primary goal of ACLS is early defibrillation.

Ref I: page 2215

2. Answer . . . a.

This is a true statement. When this ECG sign exists, the patient is presumed to be myocardially infarcting.

Ref I: page 2211

3. Answer . . . b.

Diltiazem has a negative inotropic effect. Nitroprusside produces vasodilatation. Please refer to the cardiogenic shock/acute pulmonary edema algorithm for recommendations regarding management of the hypotensive patient with signs and symptoms of pump failure.

Ref I: pages 2226–2228

4. Answer . . . b

Atropine is employed initially until capture can be achieved with TCP. A dopamine drip should also be prepared as a backup while the patient is prepared for a *transvenous* pacemaker.

Ref I: pages 2221–2222

5. Answer . . . b.

Endotracheal intubation is a class I (definitely helpful) intervention during cardiac arrest for all the reasons listed. It is not indicated in those whose airway can be maintained noninvasively.

Ref I: pages 2201–2203

6. Answer . . . a.

Versatile bag–valve devices can be used with masks and with ET tubes to deliver 100% oxygen. A second rescuer is advisable when bag–valve–mask ventilation is required, as leaks around the mask are a common problem. In some studies mouth-to-mask ventilation achieved greater tidal volumes.

Ref I: pages 2199–2200

7. Answer . . . b.

The mainstay of acid–base management during cardiac arrest is hyperventilation and CPR. In prolonged arrest, sodium bicarbonate is possibly helpful (class IIb) *only* if the patient is intubated. Because this drug releases CO_2, acidosis may worsen with its use.

Ref I pages 2210–2211

8. Answer . . . d.

Suctioning through an ET tube must be performed using flexible sterile tracheal suction catheters. Attempts should not exceed 15 seconds. The high potential for arrhythmias and hypoxia demands hyperoxygenation before and in between attempts.

Ref II: Chapter 2, page 15

9. Answer . . . d.

An intubated cardiac arrest victim can be hyperventilated using large tidal volumes. Because adult resuscitation units do not have pop-off valves, ventilation need not be synchronized with compressions.

Ref I: pages 2201–2202

10. Answer . . . d.

Simultaneously with the delivery of the first manual breath, the epigastrium should be auscultated. If gurgling is heard and the chest does not rise, esophageal intubation can be assumed.

Ref I: page 2202

11. Answer . . . c.

This simple device allows the operator to customize ET tube curvature to conform to individual upper airway shapes. For safety reasons, the end of the stylet must be recessed 1/2 inch from the tip of the tube.

Ref II: Chapter 2, page 4

12. Answer . . . a.

Requiring a second rescuer, cricoid pressure not only helps prevent aspiration of gastric contents, but assists alignment of the axis of the upper airways.

Ref II: Chapter 2, pages 4–5

13. Answer . . . b.

Operator shock from these devices is not a hazard. Poor patient tolerance does, however, often necessitate sedation. TCP is invaluable in providing patient stabilization until a transvenous pacemaker (TVP) can be placed.

Ref II: Chapter 5, pages 2–5

14. Answer . . . b.

Atrial flutter and PSVT often convert at this lower energy level. Please refer to the electrical cardioversion algorithm.

Ref I: pages 2223–2225

15. Answer . . . d.

All of these factors should be considered to provide lower transthoracic impedance.

Ref I: page 2212

16. Answer . . . a.

This potent inotrope possesses no vasopressor action. Therefore, increases in BP are due to higher cardiac output. Tachycardic side effects can be pronounced at higher doses.

Ref I: page 2209

17. Answer . . . c.

As the stable tachycardia algorithm illustrate; a lidocaine–lidocaine–adenosine–adenosine–procainamide–bretylium sequence is indicated for these rhythms.

Ref I: page 2223

18. Answer . . . a.

Isoproterenol has earned widespread disfavor due to its adverse effect on ischemia and infarct size. It is a class III (harmful) intervention at higher doses and a class IIb (possibly helpful) intervention at lower doses.

Ref I: page 2222

19. Answer . . . c.

Administration of verapamil to a patient with VT can be a lethal error. Accordingly, the stable tachycardia algorithm is designed to prohibit administration of this agent to all wide-complex rhythms.

Ref I: pages 2223–2225

20. Answer . . . a.

The acute myocardial infarction algorithm illustrates the host of actions that are indicated in managing the patient with uncomplicated AMI.

Ref I: pages 2230–2232; Ref II: Chapter 1, pages 47–58

21. Answer . . . a.

Epinephrine is a definitely helpful (class I) agent for all forms of cardiac arrest. A volume infusion is indicated as is the rapid search for treatable causes. Atropine is not indicated unless a bradyarrhythmia exists.

Ref I: pages 2219–2220

22. Answer . . . b.

Third-degree AV block usually relies on an idioventricular escape focus to capture the ventricles. Unless treatment is prompt, idioventricular rhythms tend to become progressively bradyasystolic, and finally deteriorate to complete asystole.

Ref I: page 2222

23. Answer . . . a.

Because cannulation requires interruption of CPR, central veins are not used unless previous access exists. Because of their proximity to large arteries and the lungs, their use is associated with the complications described.

Ref II: Chapter 6, pages 1–2

24. Answer . . . b.

When used in cardiac arrest, the initial dosage of sodium bicarbonate is 1 mEq/kg. Half that dosage may be given every ten minutes thereafter.

Ref I: pages 2210–2211

25. Answer . . . d.

As defibrillation is the only definitive therapy for VF/VT, it is indicated even if the interval between arrest and the first shocks is prolonged.

Ref I: pages 2215–2217

26. Answer . . . c.

Norepinephrine is indicated for cardiogenic shock that does not respond to dopamine. The patient with uncomplicated AMI should be supported with oxygen, morphine, nitroglycerin, an IV line, and cardiac monitoring.

Ref I: pages 2230–2231

27. Answer . . . d.

If endotracheal drug administration is indicated, medications should be administered at 2.0 to 2.5 times the recommended IV dose and should be diluted in 10 mL of normal saline or distilled water.

Ref I: page 2205

28. Answer . . . d.

Atropine is a parasympatholytic agent that is useful in treating bradyarrhythmias. It may result in increased myocardial oxygen demand. For this reason, it must be used cautiously in patients with acute ischemic heart disease.

Ref I: page 2207

29. Answer . . . d.

This beneficial agent produces vasodilatory hemodynamic effects that reduce infarct size when used in the setting of possible AMI. Its mainstay status is confirmed by the hundreds of thousands of patients who employ it successfully to manage angina.

Ref I: page 2210

30. Answer . . . d.

Sodium bicarbonate is a class IIa (probably helpful) agent when cardiac arrest is due to pre-existing acidosis, and tricyclic over-dose. It is considered harmful (class III) in the management of the hypoxic lactic acidosis associated with cardiac arrest. It is a IIb (possibly helpful) agent in prolonged cardiac arrest with intubation.

Ref I: page 2210

31. Answer . . . b.

According to the VF/VT algorithm, after three initial attempts at defibrillation, airway and IV access are to be obtained. Epinephrine can then be administered and, if necessary, followed by a defibrillatory attempt at 360 J.

Ref I: pages 2215–2217

32. Answer . . . c.

According to the VF/VT algorithm, the correct sequence is depicted in choice c.

Ref I: pages 2215–2217

33. Answer . . . d.

When faced with a "flatline" on the monitor, rescuers should obtain confirmation by changing to another lead or by rotating defibrillator paddles 90°. Operator error is reportedly much more common than is isoelectric VF.

Ref I: page 2220

34. Answer . . . a.

Hemodynamic instability is typically manifested by a systolic BP less than 80 mm Hg in the presence of confirming signs and symptoms. Unstable tachycardias must be treated with synchronized cardioversion.

Ref I: pages 2222–2224

35. Answer . . . b.

The stable tachycardia algorithm indicates that after two doses of adenosine, rhythm width and BP can be assessed. If the complex is narrow and the BP is not low, verapamil 2.5 to 5 mg is indicated.

Ref I: pages 2222–2224

36. Answer . . . a.

Lidocaine is not indicated in the setting of possible AMI accompanied by asymptomatic PVCs. In this context, ectopy is a warning that ischemia exists and needs specific treatment. Signs of ischemia should not be masked with antiarrhythmic drugs.

Ref II: Chapter 1, page 58

37. Answer . . . b.

Second-degree type II and third-degree rhythms with infranodal block are potentially lethal arrhythmias. Preparation should begin immediately for a transvenous pacemaker. Atropine and TCP can be used to provide stability until a TVP is placed.

Ref I: pages 2221–2222

38. Answer . . . c.

As electrical therapy is present, the synchronizer switch should be turned off and defibrillation performed immediately.

Ref I: pages 2217–2220

39. Answer . . . d.

After noting the presence of pulselessness and VF, the rescuer should call for a defibrillator and perform CPR until its arrival.

Ref I: pages 2217–2220

40. Answer . . . d.

Multiple signs and symptoms confirm the presence of an unstable tachycardia. Synchronized countershocks at 50 J to 100 J is indicated. Verapamil is contraindicated in all wide-complex tachycardias.

Ref I: pages 2224–2225

41. Answer . . . d.

In addition to CPR and epinephrine, rescuers must search for treatable underlying causes by evaluating the patient as indicated in question 41. Blood flow can be assessed with Doppler or end-tidal CO_2 monitoring devices.

Ref III: Chapter 9, pages 4-1–4-12

42. Answer . . . d.

Lidocaine and a fluid challenge are not part of the routine management of uncomplicated AMI.

Ref II: Chapter 1, pages 47–58

43. Answer . . . d.

Atropine is the IV agent of initial choice. Isoproterenol is the agent of least choice. Epinephrine is generally administered only if the patient cannot be stabilized with dopamine.

Ref I: pages 2221–2222

44. Answer . . . b.

Patients who are older than 70 years of age and those with symptoms lasting longer than six hours present *relative* contraindications to thrombolytic therapy that would have to be weighed carefully by medical personnel.

Ref II: Chapter 1, pages 51–52

45. Answer . . . d.

All of these factors provide clues which suggest the presence of cardiac tamponade. Recent evidence of an enlarged heart shadow on x-ray and pulsus paradoxus would provide further evidence. If the patient is in life-threatening distress, emergency pericardiocentesis is indicated.

Ref III: Chapter 9, pages 4–5, 4–6

46. Answer . . . d.

Sodium bicarbonate cannot be administered via the ET tube. Only lipid-soluble drugs such as atropine, lidocaine, epinephrine, and naloxone can be administered via this route.

Ref I: page 2267

47. Answer . . . d.

During cardiac arrest, obtaining IV access without interrupting CPR is of necessity a greater concern than strict asepsis. In an emergency, practical considerations are foremost.

Ref II: Chapter 5, pages 1–9

48. Answer . . . b.

Slowing the ventricular rate is the goal of pharmacologic therapy in treating atrial fibrillation. To do this, drugs must be used that increase the refractoriness of the AV node. Calcium channel blockers, beta-blocking agents, and digitalis are useful in this regard.

Ref I: page 2224

49. Answer . . . c.

For a patient with signs and symptoms of acute pulmonary edema without hemodynamic instability, a vasopressor agent such as dopamine is not indicated. Morphine and nitroglycerin provide useful hemodynamic actions for the patient with APE. Furosemide is an old standby that must be used with caution in patients with systolic BPs less than 100 mm Hg.

Ref II: Chapter 1, pages 40–46

50. Answer . . . c.

After activating an AED device's analysis mode, the absence of VF/VT will result in a "no shock indicated" command. This does not mean cardiac arrest does not exist! Remember, AEDs are attached only to pulseless patients. The victim may be pulseless due to a nonshockable rhythm. To make this determination, you must check the pulse.

Ref II: Chapter 4, pages 8–11

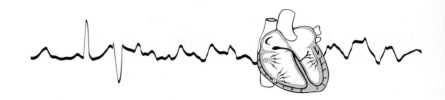

1. ACLS Course Requirements

THE ACLS EDUCATIONAL PROCESS

In 1992, the American Heart Association (AHA), published its latest guidelines for providing adult advanced cardiac life support (ACLS). These recommendations appeared in the *Journal of the American Medical Association* (*JAMA*) in its October 28, 1992 issue. Subsequently, the AHA subcommittees in ACLS and electrocardiography (ECG) met to design a training program to best teach these guidelines. The results of this educational conference were published in May of 1994.

Your ACLS provider course is built around recommendations that were advanced by the ACLS Educational Task Force in their 1994 conference proceedings. Some of these recommendations reflect a refocusing of previous educational goals. Others, such as the switch to case-based education, are considered a departure.

Briefly, the most important of these recommendations are as follows.

ACLS Courses Train Providers: They Do *Not* Certify Competence

Your ACLS course is an educational tool for health care providers whose workplace activities require proficiency in the management of cardiac arrest. Individuals who satisfactorily complete an ACLS course are termed

"ACLS providers." Completion of the course does *not* imply the granting of any "certificate," "license," or other "warranty" of competence.

The Primary Goal of ACLS Programs Is Restated

ACLS courses are designed to enhance the skills and knowledge of participants in providing resuscitative efforts to patients in cardiac arrest.

ACLS Testing Is an Educational Tool

To successfully complete an ACLS course, participants must undergo an evaluation process. The purpose of this testing is to identify areas of weakness so that course participants and instructors can focus their efforts on improvement of skills and knowledge.

"Harmful Stress" Must Be Eliminated From Courses

Course directors and instructors are reminded that the purpose of ACLS training is to educate. Their responsibility is to *facilitate* that process. "Reasonable remediation" should be the instructor's primary response to areas of weakness that are identified.

The instructor is not responsible for *certifying* that a level of proficiency exists. Therefore, the threat of course failure is not appropriate and does not have a place in the ACLS educational process.

An ACLS Course Is Not a Pharmacology or an Arrhythmia Course

Time does not permit more than a brief *review* of those subjects. Course participants who lack expertise are strongly advised to complete refresher courses in these areas *prior* to participation in an ACLS program.

ACLS Courses Must Use *Case-based* NOT *Subject-based* Teaching

Prior to 1994, adult ACLS courses were built around lectures on traditional subjects such as pharmacology, arrhythmia recognition, acute myocardial infarction, etc. Following these lectures, participants were asked to demonstrate these subject-based skills in various stations. Thus, airways and intubation were demonstrated at one station, and defibrillation at yet another. Thus, while competence in a given subject area was measured, there was no assurance that course participants could "put it all together" and manage or problem solve cases typical of adult ACLS.

In current *case-based* ACLS courses, participants manage nine different patient care scenarios, each of which can be varied to meet individual backgrounds and needs.

Because the emphasis is on "ACLS management" of a given case, course participants must be prepared to demonstrate *all* relevant skills as the scenario develops.

For example, in any given case, participants may be asked to perform cardiopulmonary resuscitation (CPR), manage the airway, assure IV access, interpret the ECG, and finally, after evaluating the patient's hemodynamic status, implement appropriate interventions. The instructor can change the patient's signs and symptoms or their response to therapy in any number of ways to best suit the needs of the student. The advantages of this approach are considerable for both course participant and instructor.

TYPES OF ACLS COURSES

The "Essentials of ACLS" Course

Designed for less experienced providers, these courses cover only the nine "core" or "essential" ACLS cases.

Each one of these is built around a specific ACLS algorithm. These algorithms appear in Chapter 13, The ACLS Cases. Chapter 13 also details the critical performance skills required to demonstrate proficiency. These algorithms also appear in the chapters on airways (Chapter 3), electrical therapy (Chapter 4), pharmacology (Chapter 9), and arrhythmia recognition (Chapters 10, 11, and 12).

Please be aware, once again, that *only* these nine algorithms and their respective cases are taught as part of an Essentials of ACLS course. These nine essential ACLS cases and their algorithms are listed below:

- Case 1: Respiratory Arrest with a Pulse/The Universal Algorithm
- Case 2: Witnessed Adult Cardiac Arrest/The Automated External Defibrillator Algorithm
- Case 3: Mega VF–Refractory VF/VT/The VF/VT Algorithm
- Case 4: Pulseless Electrical Activity/The Pulseless Electrical Activity Algorithm
- Case 5: Asystole/The Asystole Algorithm
- Case 6: Acute Myocardial Infarction/The Acute Myocardial Infarction Algorithm
- Case 7: Bradycardia/The Bradycardia Algorithm
- Case 8: Unstable Tachycardia/The Electrical Cardioversion Algorithm
- Case 9: Stable Tachycardia/The Stable Tachycardia Algorithm

The "Comprehensive" ACLS Course

Designed for more experienced providers such as physicians, these courses are designed to cover "noncore" or "supplemental" material. This material is evaluated as part of nine supplemental ACLS cases. These cases are listed below.

- Case 10: Hypotension/Shock/Acute Pulmonary Edema
- Case 11: Cardiac Arrest Due to Drowning
- Case 12: Hypothermia
- Case 13: Cardiac Arrest Due to Trauma
- Case 14: Cardiac Arrest Due to Electrical Shock
- Case 15: Acute Stroke
- Case 16: ACLS Ethics
- Case 17: Psychological Aspects of Resuscitation
- Case 18: Phased Response Resuscitation

Because these cases are not part of an Essentials of ACLS course, they will *not* be taught as part of this review text.

Course Length

Most ACLS courses are designed to be two days or 16 hours in length. This format usually allows time for only a brief review of complex subjects such as rhythm recognition and pharmacology.

One-day or 8-hour courses may be offered to more experienced providers such as those who provide defibrillation, IV access, rhythm recognition, and intubation as part of the daily requirements of their workplace.

CURRICULA FOR AN "ESSENTIALS OF ACLS" COURSE

Case-specific Curricula

According to the American Heart Association's *Instructor's Manual for Advanced Cardiac Life Support*, the nine essential ACLS cases are designed to evaluate the knowledge and skills detailed below. Course instructors and directors are required to cover each of the competencies listed. At the same time, they are urged to be flexible and to tailor these cases to meet the needs of individual students.

Case 1: Respiratory Arrest With a Pulse (*Airway Adjuncts, Endotracheal Intubation, IV Access*)

- Understanding of the Universal Algorithm
- Insertion of oropharyngeal and nasopharyngeal airways
- Barrier devices
- Bag–valve–mask ventilation
- Mouth-to-mask ventilation
- Oxygen administration devices (nasal cannulas, face masks, nonrebreathing masks)
- Endotracheal intubation and its complications

- Peripheral IV access and its complications
- Pharyngeal suctioning and its complications

Case 2: Witnessed Ventricular Fibrillation (VF)

- Understanding of the universal algorithm
- Noninvasive airway management skills
- Oxygen administration devices
- CPR: one and two person
- Operation and use of AEDs (automated external defibrillators)
- Post resuscitation management

Case 3: Mega-Ventricular Fibrillation: Refractory Ventricular Fibrillation

- Team leader role
- Team member role
- Rhythm recognition skills
- Defibrillation with conventional defibrillators
- Defibrillation safety
- Understanding of the ventricular fibrillation/ventricular tachycardia (VF/VT) algorithm
- Medications of probable and possible benefit

Case 4: Pulseless Electrical Activity

- Team leader role
- Team member role
- Rhythm recognition skills
- Safety considerations
- Evaluation of patient to determine underlying cause
- Universal algorithm
- Understanding of the pulseless electrical activity algorithm
- Cardiac tamponade
- Tension pneumothorax
- Hypovolemia
- Hypoxia

Case 5: Asystole

- Team leader role
- Team member role
- Rhythm recognition skills
- Understanding of the asystole algorithm
- Evaluation of patient to determine underlying cause
- The role of external pacing
- Maintenance of acid–base balance
- Termination of efforts

Case 6: Acute Myocardial Infarction (AMI)

- Understanding of the AMI algorithm
- Community approach to ACLS
- Emergency medical services (EMS) protocols
- Emergency department approach to ACLS
- Rapid "door-to-treatment" interval
- Indications and contraindications for thrombolytic therapy
- Major drugs to consider in AMI
- Recognition of acute ischemia and injury on ECG

Case 7: Unstable Bradycardia

- Rhythm recognition skills
- Understanding of the unstable bradycardia algorithm
- External pacing
- Major drugs to consider
- Concept of "symptomatic" bradycardia

Case 8: Unstable Tachycardia

- Rhythm recognition skills
- Understanding of the unstable tachycardia algorithm
- Understanding of the synchronized cardioversion algorithm
- Major drugs to consider
- Concept of "stable" tachycardia

Case 9: Stable Tachycardia

- Rhythm recognition skills
- Understanding of the stable tachycardia algorithm
- Major drugs to consider
- Concept of "symptomatic" tachycardia

Core Pharmacology and Rhythm Recognition Curricula

According to the current AHA *Instructor's Manual for Advanced Cardiac Life Support*, ACLS course participants are required to demonstrate proficiency in rhythm recognition and administration of pharmacologic agents. The following competencies are designated therein as being part of an Essentials of ACLS course.

Core ACLS Pharmacology Curricula

For each of the therapeutic interventions or options listed below, ACLS course participants must demonstrate an understanding of the following therapeutic principles as they relate to ACLS.

- Mechanisms of action (why?)
- Indications (when?)
- Dosage (how?)
- Hazards and Precautions
  IV fluids
  Oxygen
  Epinephrine
  Lidocaine
  Bretylium
  Magnesium sulfate
  Procainamide
  Sodium bicarbonate
  Atropine
  Dopamine
  Isoproterenol
  Vagal maneuvers (used as a drug)
  Adenosine
  Verapamil
  Diltiazem
  Beta blockers (eg, atenolol, propanolol, esmolol, or metoprolol)
  Nitroglycerin
  Nitroprusside
  Dobutamine
  Morphine sulfate
  Furosemide
  A thrombolytic agent (the one used in provider's work setting)
  Defibrillation
  Cardioversion
  Transcutaneous pacing

Essential ACLS Rhythm Recognition Skills

ACLS course participants must be able to recognize the following core arrhythmias. In addition, they must be able to demonstrate an understanding of the intervention sequence recommended for each in the nine ACLS algorithms.

- Lethal arrhythmias
  VF/pulseless VT
  Asystole
  Pulseless electrical activity
  Electrocardiographic artifact
- The bradycardias
  Sinus bradycardia
  Junctional rhythms
  First-degree atrioventricular (AV) block
  Second-degree type I AV block
  Third-degree AV block

- The tachycardias
  Sinus tachycardia
  Atrial flutter
  Atrial fibrillation
  Paroxysmal supraventricular tachycardia (PSVT)
  Atrial tachycardia with block
  Premature ventricular contractions (PVCs)
  Ventricular tachycardia
  Torsade de pointes/polymorphic VT
  Wide-complex tachycardias of uncertain origin
- Electrocardiographic indications for thrombolytic therapy
  Signs of myocardial ischemia
  Signs of myocardial injury/infarcting status
  Signs of myocardial infarction

BIBLIOGRAPHY

1. American Heart Association, Emergency Cardiac Care Committee and Subcommittees. Guidelines for cardiopulmonary resuscitation and emergency cardiac care. JAMA 1992;268:2171–2295
2. American Heart Association. Textbook of advanced cardiac life support. Dallas, TX: American Heart Association, 1994
3. American Heart Association. Instructor's manual for advanced cardiac life support. Dallas, TX: American Heart Association, 1994
4. Proceedings of the National Conference on ECC and CPR. Ann Emerg Med 1993;22(Part 2):275–511
5. Billi JE. The educational direction of the ACLS training program. Ann Emerg Med 1993;22(Part 2):484–488
6. Billi J, Membrino G. Education in adult advanced cardiac life support training programs: changing the paradigm. Ann Emerg Med 1993;22(Part 2):475–483

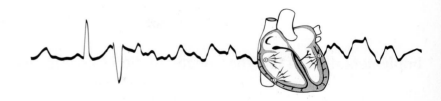

2. Principles of Adult ACLS

OUTLINE

The 1992 National Conference on CPR and ECC

What Is ACLS?

Why Is ACLS Necessary?

Risk Factors for Coronary Artery Disease

The Chain of Survival: Implementing Community-Wide ECC

ACLS Conceptual Tools

The Therapeutic Option Classification System

The Algorithm Approach to ACLS and ECC

THE 1992 NATIONAL CONFERENCE ON CPR AND ECC

In February 1992, the fifth national conference on CPR and emergency cardiac care (ECC) was held. The proceedings of that conference were published in the October 28, 1992 issue of the *Journal of the American Medical Association*. Significant areas of emphasis to come out of the conference were as follows.

Elimination of the Term "Standards" From the Conference Proceedings

Earlier conferences on CPR and ECC, held in 1974, 1979, and 1985, had employed the term "standards" to describe their scientific findings. Citing the fact that the term had acquired unwanted legal implications, it was purposely not used in the 1992 publication.

In its place, the terms *guidelines* and *recommendations* are used. The desired outcome of this action is that therapeutic options recommended not be accorded an overly firm or inflexible clinical status.

Implementation of the Therapeutic Option Classification System

After carefully weighing existing scientific evidence, therapeutic interventions were given scaled recommendations using the following four-point classification system:

- Class I: Definitely helpful
- Class IIa: Probably helpful
- Class IIb: Possibly helpful
- Class III: May be harmful

Implementing the Algorithm Approach to ECC

The conference proceedings as published in the October 28, 1992 issue of *JAMA* strongly emphasize the educational nature of the ACLS algorithms. These guidelines state that they "must be used wisely, not blindly." The guidelines further encourage flexibility in their use when clinically appropriate.

Endorsement of the Early Use of Thrombolytic Agents in AMI

Citing dramatic improvements in outcome reported by some centers, the 1992 *JAMA* guidelines give thrombolytic agents a class I recommendation for patients less than 70 years of age, whose symptoms are less than six hours in duration, who have no absolute and few relative contraindications to this procedure.

Continued Endorsement of the Early Use of Defibrillation

Approximately 80 to 90% of all nontraumatic adult cardiac arrests are the result of ventricular fibrillation/pulseless ventricular tachycardia (VF/VT). Defibrillation remains the only definitive therapy for this arrhythmia. Of the 500,000 or so victims who die each year of acute myocardial infarction, roughly two-thirds expire before they reach the hospital.

The JAMA guidelines strongly support efforts to employ rapid defibrillation, particularly in the prehospital setting.

The placement of automated external defibrillators (AEDs) throughout the community, along with the training of large numbers of people in their use, is an intervention that is given their strongest endorsement.

WHAT IS ACLS?

Adult ACLS is a constellation of knowledge and skills to ensure early treatment for cardiac and respiratory arrest. Roughly 80 to 90% of cases of non-traumatic adult cardiac arrest are due to VF/VT. Thus, the primary goal of ACLS is to provide early defibrillation. ACLS also focuses on the hour or so prior to possible sudden death, as well as on providing stabilization in the postresuscitation phase.

ACLS is comprised of the following core competencies, as well as the judgmental skills necessary to safely implement them:

- Basic life support (BLS)
- Early defibrillation
- Airway maintenance, oxygenation, and ventilation
- Provision of IV access
- Synchronized cardioversion and transcutaneous pacing
- ECG monitoring and arrhythmia recognition
- Pharmacologic therapy
- Emergency management of patients with acute MI
- Management of cardiopulmonary emergencies

WHY IS ACLS NECESSARY?

Sudden death from acute myocardial infarction is the most serious public health problem in the United States. There are approximately two million deaths each year in the United States. Roughly one million of these are due to cardiovascular disease.

Acute myocardial infarction (AMI) alone is responsible for 500,000 of these deaths. Stroke is a distant second, accounting for approximately 150,000 deaths per year. Of the half a million AMI-related deaths, roughly two-thirds occur *prior* to hospitalization, usually within 2 hours after onset of symptoms. Further analysis of these victims has revealed the following information:

- Over one-third of these heart attacks occur in victims less than 65 years of age.
- In up to 20% of cardiac arrest victims, sudden death is the first evidence of cardiovascular disease.
- The majority of victims of sudden arrhythmic death experience no premonitoring symptoms immediately prior to collapse.

It is an extraordinary fact that one quarter of the annual deaths in the United States are due to thrombotic occlusion of just two of the body's innumerable blood vessels. Furthermore, 80 to 90% of adult cardiac arrests are precipitated by VF/VT, a rhythm that is highly amenable to early defibrillation.

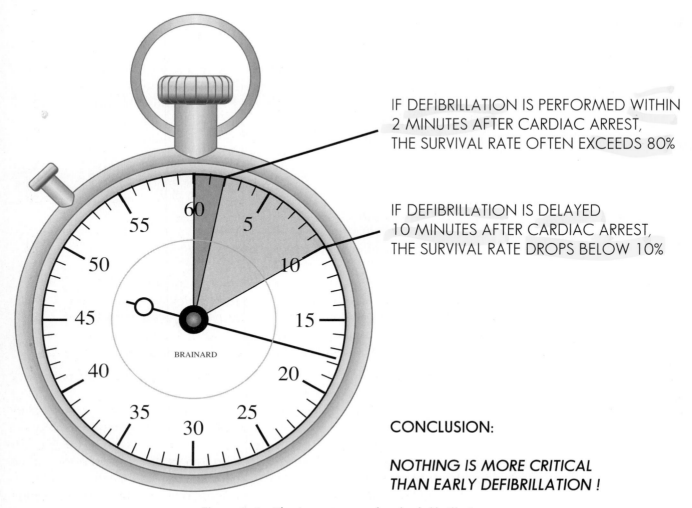

IF DEFIBRILLATION IS PERFORMED WITHIN 2 MINUTES AFTER CARDIAC ARREST, THE SURVIVAL RATE OFTEN EXCEEDS 80%

IF DEFIBRILLATION IS DELAYED 10 MINUTES AFTER CARDIAC ARREST, THE SURVIVAL RATE DROPS BELOW 10%

CONCLUSION:

NOTHING IS MORE CRITICAL THAN EARLY DEFIBRILLATION !

Figure 2–1. The importance of early defibrillation.

As a consequence, the *cornerstone* of ACLS and its primary goal is the provision of early defibrillation. It is not possible to overstate the importance of early defibrillation on improved outcomes. No other intervention is associated with greater likelihood of survival.

Figure 2–1 illustrates the importance of early defibrillation. For a more detailed discussion of the principles of defibrillation, please refer to Chapter 4 in this review text.

RISK FACTORS FOR CORONARY ARTERY DISEASE

Mortality from cardiovascular disease, including AMI and stroke, has been dropping significantly over the past three decades. Since the mid-1960s, the decline has averaged between 2 and 3% each year. Several factors related to advances in medical treatment and healthier lifestyles are responsible for this improving picture.

Identification of Patients at High Risk

In roughly 20% of cardiac arrest victims, sudden death is the first evidence of coronary artery disease. Attempts to identify these individuals is an important goal of the American Heart Association and other community health organizations.

Persons with a family history of cardiovascular disease and those with diabetes mellitus must be made aware that they are at risk for AMI.

Although trauma is the leading cause of death in individuals less than 44 years of age, these individuals must be made aware that they too are at risk if their lifestyle does not include regular exercise, weight control, cessation of smoking, and control of blood pressure.

Reducing Risk Factors

Gender, age, race, and *heredity* are risk factors that cannot be modified. Other factors can be changed and it is best to do so at a young age. Nevertheless, positive impact can be obtained even when intervention is delayed until later in life. The following factors are of particular importance:

- **Cigarette smoking.** Cigarette smoking is the single most important cause of preventable death in the United States.
- **Hypertension.** In recent years, there has been striking improvement in the management of this risk factor. A systolic blood pressure (BP) greater than 160 mm Hg or a diastolic BP greater than 95 mm Hg is associated with a two- to threefold increase in the risk of coronary artery disease.
- **Cholesterol.** The Framingham Study has shown that the ratio of total cholesterol to high-density cholesterol is a good tool to predict the risk for coronary artery disease in the asymptomatic individual. Efforts at dietary and pharmacologic control are expected to have proportionate impact on reduction of mortality from coronary artery disease.
- **Lack of exercise.** Regular physical exercise is strongly associated with reduced risk for coronary artery disease.
- **Obesity.** Obesity is associated with hypertension, diabetes, and elevated cholesterol.
- **Stress.** Chronic stress, and the extent to which stressful lifestyle is related to coronary artery disease, has proved difficult to measure. However, stress reduction techniques *have* been shown to help control hypertension.

THE CHAIN OF SURVIVAL: IMPLEMENTING COMMUNITY-WIDE ECC

Once cardiac arrest or other signs and symptoms of AMI have occurred, a sequence of urgent critical actions must be accomplished if a successful outcome is to be achieved.

The JAMA guidelines refer to this concept as the "chain of survival." It is composed of four interdependent links, each of which is an essential component of the community-wide ECC system, as described below.

- **The first link: Early access.** Access to the community ECC system is obtained by dialing 911. Trained *dispatchers* must then send EMS personnel to provide care. Inherent problems in obtaining early access include:
  - Patient denial of symptoms. An unacceptable 3 to 4 hours often lapses between the onset of symptoms and dialing of 911.
  - Urban and rural settings. EMS responders are often delayed by urban traffic. Similar delays are encountered when large distances must be traversed in rural settings.
- **The second link: Early CPR.** Bystander CPR has been shown to have a positive effect on survival. Community-wide CPR programs are strongly encouraged by the AHA. However, because 80 to 90% of all nontraumatic adult cardiac arrests are due to VF/VT, CPR *alone* is of limited value.
- **The third link: Early defibrillation.** Early defibrillation is the "strongest link in the chain of survival." The reason is clear: Only defibrillation provides definitive treatment for VF/VT. When performed within two minutes, survival rates as high as 80% are noted. Defibrillation can be achieved by use of automated or conventional devices. The JAMA guidelines state that both methods are equally effective.
- **The fourth link: Early ACLS.** Community EMS systems should provide *paramedic responders* who are trained in ACLS. These individuals can, in addition to providing rapid defibrillation, provide airway and IV access, administer drugs, and identify and treat cardiac arrhythmias.

ACLS CONCEPTUAL TOOLS

Many ACLS providers have a vast reservoir of experience from which to draw, having participated in or conducted hundreds of codes. In emergencies, they function quickly and effectively. For them, going through the "ABCs" has become instinct.

The American Heart Association's textbook of ACLS and instructor's manual utilize two conceptual frameworks as tools to guide less experienced providers through their ACLS performance stations. Both provide systems which can be applied to the diverse nature of ACLS.

The Primary/Secondary ABCD Surveys

Although designed to be utilized for patients in cardiac arrest, the *primary/secondary approach* can be applied to virtually any emergency situation. To the novice, applying the principles of ACLS (rhythms, drugs,

IVs, airways, etc.) to a wide variety of patients seems like an impossible task. Not without reason does the expert make it look as easy as "ABCD"!

The Primary Survey

- Determine unresponsiveness/call for help
- **A**irway
  Open the airway
- **B**reathing
  Look, listen, feel
  Give two slow breaths pausing in between
- **C**irculation
  Assess pulselessness
  Begin CPR
- **D**efibrillation
  Attach monitor/defibrillator
  Perform immediate defibrillation if VF/VT is present

The Secondary Survey

- **A**irway
  Perform endotracheal intubation if indicated
  Secure the airway using noninvasive techniques if indicated
- **B**reathing
  Determine proper placement of the endotracheal tube
  Provide adequacy of ventilation using bag-valve or other positive-pressure device
- **C**irculation
  Obtain IV access
  Attach ECG monitor leads
  Identify rhythm and rate
  Monitor blood pressure
  Provide medications appropriate for cardiac rate, rhythm, and blood pressure
- **D**ifferential **D**iagnosis
  During each code effort, team members should employ a *systematic differential diagnosis* process to help determine the underlying causes of the cardiopulmonary emergency. ACLS providers are encouraged to think beyond traditional rhythm, BP, and rate-specific therapeutic interventions. Many of the patients requiring this in-depth approach will be ones who do not respond to defibrillation, or who have asystole or pulseless electrical activity (PEA). For most of these victims, unless a *treatable underlying cause* is promptly found, code efforts will have been in vain.

The Four Triads

This conceptual tool can be used in any patient who is *not* in cardiac arrest. Like the primary/secondary approach, it is easily remembered. It is as follows:

1. Airway–Breathing–Circulation
2. Oxygen–IV–Monitor
3. Pulse–Respiration–Blood Pressure
4. Rate Problem–Pump Problem–Volume Problem

These triads provide a logical framework for initial management of patients who are both hemodynamically stable and unstable.

THE THERAPEUTIC OPTION CLASSIFICATION SYSTEM

One of the more important developments to come out of the 1992 National Conference on CPR and ECC was its attempt to classify the effectiveness of drugs and other therapeutic modalities used during CPR. Accordingly, conference committee and subcommittee participants were asked to weigh the scientific evidence regarding each therapeutic intervention.

Evaluation criteria for scientific data was constructed so that only those studies adhering to strict research and scientific principles would be acceptable. The criteria were as follows:

* Random placebo-controlled studies were preferred.
* Studies blinded to intervention weighted most heavily.
* Studies utilizing clinically relevant methods were preferred, as were those with a sample size large enough to minimize error.
* Results were considered most valid if similar conclusions were reached by separate groups of investigators.
* Finally, the ethical content of the study had to be considered commensurate with acceptable clinical practice, *especially* concerning informed consent.

Using these criteria, the conference participants were able to classify most therapeutic interventions as to whether they fit into one of the following four well-defined categories:

* Class I: *Definitely* helpful
  Interventions in this category are usually indicated, always acceptable, and considered useful and effective.
* Class IIa: *Probably* helpful
  Interventions in this category have the weight of evidence in favor of its usefulness and efficiency.
* Class IIb: *Possibly* helpful
  The intervention is not well established by evidence but *may* be helpful and probably is not harmful.

- Class III: May be *harmful*
  The therapeutic option is inappropriate, is without scientific supporting data, and may be harmful.

THE ALGORITHM APPROACH TO ACLS AND ECC

Another important feature of the 1992 National Conference on CPR and ECC was the development of the essential and supplemental ACLS algorithms.

The JAMA guidelines assert that these algorithms were designed for educational and illustrative value only. Further, they warn, because it is their nature to oversimplify, they must be "used wisely and not blindly." ACLS providers are encouraged to be flexible in employing them as long as clinical appropriateness is assured. Finally, the guidelines caution that the algorithms not be considered "endorsements, requirements, or standards of care in a legal sense."

The following recommendations apply to all ACLS algorithms:

- First, *treat the patient, not the monitor.*
- Algorithms for cardiac arrest presume that the condition under discussion continually persists, that the patient remains in cardiac arrest, and that CPR is always performed.
- Apply different interventions whenever appropriate indications exist.
- The flow diagrams present mostly class I (acceptable, definitely effective) recommendations. The footnotes present class IIa (acceptable, probably effective), class IIb (acceptable, possibly effective), and class III (not indicated, may be harmful) recommendations.
- Adequate airway, ventilation, oxygenation, chest compressions, and defibrillation are more important than administration of medications and *take precedence* over initiating an intravenous line or injecting pharmacologic agents.
- Several medications (epinephrine, lidocaine, and atropine) can be administered via the endotracheal tube, but clinicians must use an endotracheal dose 2 to 2.5 times the intravenous dose.
- With a few exceptions, intravenous medications should be administered rapidly, in bolus method.
- After each intravenous medication, give a 20- to 30-mL bolus of intravenous fluid and *immediately* elevate the extremity. This will enhance delivery of drugs to the central circulation.
- Last, *treat the patient, not the monitor.*

BIBLIOGRAPHY

1. American Heart Association, Emergency Cardiac Care Committee and Subcommittees. Guidelines for cardiopulmonary resuscitation and emergency cardiac care. JAMA 1992;268:2171–2295

2. American Heart Association. Textbook of advanced cardiac life support. Dallas, TX: American Heart Association, 1994

3. American Heart Association. Instructor's manual for advanced cardiac life support. Dallas, TX: American Heart Association, 1994

4. Crimmins TJ. Ethical issues in adult resuscitation. Ann Emerg Med 1993; 22(Part 2):495–501

5. Proceedings of the Second Chicago Symposium on Advances in CPR Research and Guidelines for Laboratory Research. Ann Emerg Med 1996;27:539–562

6. Sanders A. Development of AHA guidelines for emergency cardiac care. Respir Care 1995;40(4):338–345

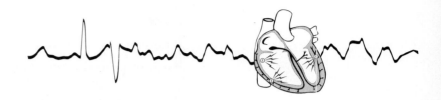

3. Endotracheal Intubation and Airway Adjuncts

OUTLINE

Essential ACLS Curricula

Role of Oxygenation and Ventilation in ACLS

The Universal Algorithm

Airway Maintenance Adjuncts

Endotracheal Intubation

Supplemental Ventilatory Adjuncts

Oxygen Administration Devices

Suctioning Devices and Techniques

Endotracheal Drug Administration

ESSENTIAL ACLS CURRICULA

Listed below are the essential airway management intubation-related skills needed for ACLS course completion. These are assessed both on the ACLS written examination and in the patient care scenarios. Case 1: Respiratory Arrest With a Pulse, is designed to measure these competencies. These specific skills are listed below. Only material so designated is evaluated in an essentials of ACLS course.

- **Essential Airway Curricula**
  Rescue positioning
  Airway opening techniques
  Oropharyngeal airways
  Nasal cannulas
  Oxygen masks

Venturi masks

Barrier mask devices

Bag–valve–mask units

Suctioning devices and techniques

Endotracheal intubation

- **Supplemental Curricula for Comprehensive Courses**

Manually triggered oxygen-powered breathing devices

Esophageal obdurator airway (EOA)

Esophageal gastric tube airway (EGTA)

Pharyngotracheal lung airway (PTL)

Cricothyrotomy

Transtracheal catheter ventilation

The list of supplemental techniques deserves some discussion. EOA, EGTA, and PTL airways are still used. Nonetheless, they are associated with high levels of risk when compared to endotracheal intubation. Thus, these airways are considered class IIb or *possibly helpful* interventions. Endotracheal intubation is the method of choice for establishing an emergency airway. It is a class I or *definitely helpful* intervention. For this reason, it is positioned at the core of ACLS teachings.

ROLE OF OXYGENATION AND VENTILATION IN ACLS

The *JAMA* guidelines state that the provision of adequate oxygenation and ventilation are, along with defibrillation and chest compression, the most important components of ACLS. They take precedence over starting an IV line and administering medications. The guidelines further remind us that important medications can be administered endotracheally. Among them are *atropine, lidocaine,* and *epinephrine* (the mnemonic is ALE). To be effective however, the endotracheal (ET) dose must be 2.0 to 2.5 times the intravenous dose.

Assuring oxygenation and ventilation is a mainstay in the management of myocardial infarction and all other cardiopulmonary emergencies. Well-documented physiologic actions of these therapeutic modalities include:

Preventing Metabolic Acidosis

Tissue hypoxia leads to anaerobic metabolism. As metabolic acidosis ensues, many therapeutic modalities lose their effectiveness. ACLS stalwarts defibrillation and epinephrine are known to be less effective when myocardial acidosis exists.

Reducing Myocardial Injury

Studies analyzing the ST segment of the ECG have shown that supplemental oxygen reduces ischemic injury when administered to patients with AMI.

Treating Acidemia

Maintaining adequate alveolar ventilation is the most effective way to assure acid–base balance during cardiac arrest. Inducing respiratory alkalosis to normalize the pH is considered safer and more effective than administering sodium bicarbonate or other buffers.

THE UNIVERSAL ALGORITHM

In light of the importance the guidelines place on CPR, oxygenation, and ventilation, it is not surprising that these are the core skills evaluated in Case 1, Respiratory Arrest With a Pulse. This case is built around the universal algorithm illustrated in Figure 3–1.

In this algorithm, please note that the ACLS provider is asked to call for help *and* request a defibrillator at the same time. This reflects the fact that VF/VT is responsible for a very large proportion of cardiac arrests.

The sequential steps of basic life support (BLS) are designed to prevent, as well as treat, injury. Properly performed, each step prohibits the next intervention from taking place until it is proved necessary.

Steps of BLS relevant to the essential ACLS airway techniques are as follows:

Properly Position Both Victim and Rescuer

The victim should be supine and on a firm, flat surface. A prone victim should be rolled as a unit so that the head, shoulders, and torso are turned simultaneously. The rescuer should then kneel at the patient's side so that the airway can be assessed (see Figure 3–2).

Open the Airway

In unconscious patients the most common cause of airway obstruction is the tongue. Frequently, all that is needed to restore adequate spontaneous ventilation is proper positioning of the head and neck. These maneuvers must therefore be performed *before* any airway adjuncts are employed. The JAMA guidelines emphasize two techniques.

Head Tilt–Chin Lift Method

This is the method recommended for use on patients who are *not* suspected of head or neck injury. As illustrated in Figure 3–3, the head is tilted back by placing the palm of one hand on the victim's forehead and applying firm pressure. At the same time the chin is lifted upward with the other

Universal Algorithm for Adult
Emergency Cardiac Care

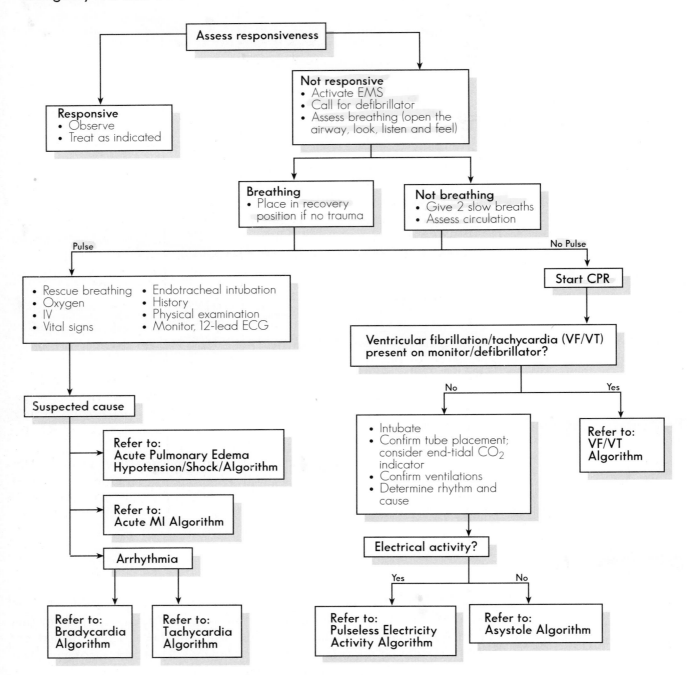

Figure 3–1. The universal algorithm for adult emergency cardiac care. The provider's understanding of this critical pathway is evaluated in Case 1, Respiratory Arrest with a Pulse. (Algorithm copyright 1992, American Medical Association; JAMA, October 28, 1992, pp 2199–2241.)

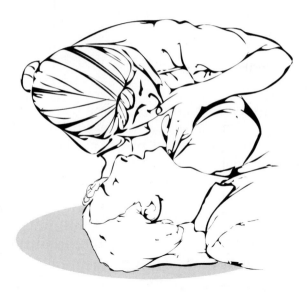

Figure 3–2. The rescuer properly positioned at the patient's side.

hand. This displaces the mandible anteriorly, lifting the tongue off the posterior pharyngeal wall.

Jaw Thrust Maneuver

Because it does not include tilting of the head, this method is not likely to extend the cervical spine. This makes it the technique of choice for patients with suspected neck injury. It is accomplished by grasping the angles of the victim's lower jaw and lifting with both hands. This action lifts the mandible upward and thus opens the airway.

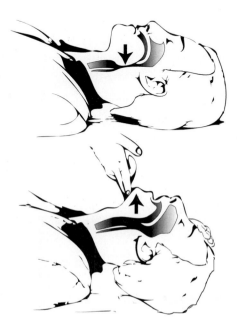

Figure 3–3. The standard head tilt–chin lift method of opening the airway.

AIRWAY MAINTENANCE ADJUNCTS

Oropharyngeal Airways

As illustrated in Figure 3–4, the oropharyngeal airway is an oval-shaped device that is hollow in the center. It is curved in such a way that it slips over the back of the tongue into the oropharynx. When placed properly, this airway prevents the tongue from occluding the upper airway.

Indications in ACLS

When used as described below, the guidelines consider the oropharyngeal airway a class I or *definitely helpful* intervention.

- To maintain the airway in *unconscious* patients with adequate spontaneous ventilation.
- To maintain the airway in nonintubated *unconscious* patients needing ventilatory assistance. Victims of cardiac arrest should be intubated promptly if defibrillation is not successful. Until an endotracheal tube can be placed, the patient must be ventilated using bag–valve–mask or mouth-to-mask techniques. To ensure adequate volume delivery with these methods, an oropharyngeal airway is recommended.

Hazards of Oropharyngeal Airways

- **Vomiting and aspiration.** These devices should *only* be used on victims who are unconscious. Gag reflex stimulation and vomiting are very real dangers and must be guarded against.

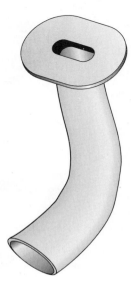

Figure 3–4. The oropharyngeal airway.

- **Improper placement.** If not properly inserted, these airways can worsen upper airway obstruction. A recommended insertion method is to turn the device so that it enters the mouth backwards. It can then be rotated as it is advanced into its proper position.
- **Use of improper size.** Oropharyngeal airways come in adult, pediatric, and neonatal sizes. The operator must learn to select the proper size for each patient. Too small an airway will not displace the tongue. Too large an airway is more likely to induce vomiting.

Nasopharyngeal Airways

As depicted in Figure 3–5, the nasopharyngeal airway is a curved rubber tube about six inches long that is designed to be placed in one nostril and passed until it lies in the posterior pharynx. Thus positioned, the device displaces the tongue and maintains airway patency.

Indications in ACLS

- Maintenance of airway patency in *conscious* or *semiconscious* victims. This airway is well tolerated in these patients and generally will not stimulate vomiting.
- Airway maintenance in patients with *trismus* who will not allow an oropharyngeal airway.

Hazards

- **Bleeding and discomfort.** Nasal tissues are both highly vascular and sensitive. Thus, care is required in placement. Topical anesthesia may be useful. Left in place too long, they can cause epistaxis on removal. Changing the airway during each shift is helpful.

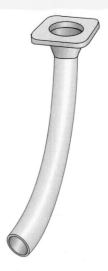

Figure 3–5. The nasopharyngeal airway.

ENDOTRACHEAL INTUBATION

Role in ACLS

As the name implies, endotracheal intubation is a procedure whereby a tube is passed into the trachea. A cuffed endotracheal tube is illustrated in Figure 3–6. Note the presence of a standard 15-mm anesthesia adaptor. The cuff, when inflated, seals off the lungs from the atmospheric gases. This allows the lungs to be ventilated, typically by a bag–valve unit. The inflated cuff also protects the lungs from aspiration of gastric contents.

The JAMA guidelines consider *orotracheal intubation* the emergency airway technique of choice during ACLS. Unfortunately, the skill required is considerable and the possibility of complications great. Thus, the guidelines stipulate, endotracheal intubation should be restricted to personnel who are specially trained and who perform the procedure frequently.

Victims of cardiac arrest require prompt intubation if initial attempts at defibrillation are not successful. For the unconscious victim without spontaneous ventilation, intubation of the trachea is considered a class I or *definitely helpful* intervention.

In contrast, the use of alternative invasive airways such as the EOA, EGTA, and PTL are considered class IIb or *possibly helpful* interventions.

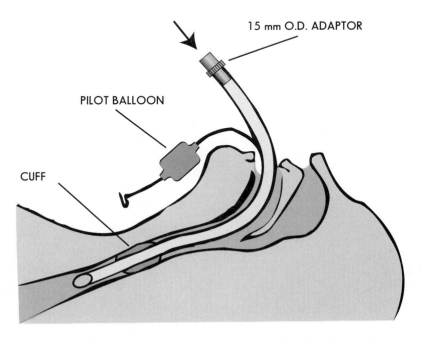

15 mm O.D. ADAPTOR

PILOT BALLOON

CUFF

Figure 3–6. Endotracheal tube in place. With its cuff inflated, ventilation can be accomplished safely and effectively.

Advantages in ACLS

- **Allows for hyperventilation.** Maintaining adequate alveolar ventilation is the most effective method of assuring acid–base balance during ACLS. Intubation allows large tidal volumes (10 to 15 mL/kg) at high rates (if necessary) to be delivered.
- **Allows drug administration.** *Atropine, lidocaine,* and *epinephrine* can be administered endotracheally. The recommended dose is 2.0 to 2.5 times the IV dose diluted in 10 mL normal saline or distilled water.
- **Allows administration of 100% oxygen.**
- **Allows for tracheal suctioning.**
- **Prevents aspiration.** When the ET tube cuff is inflated, gastric contents cannot be aspirated into the tracheobronchial tree.
- **Permits asynchronous ventilation.** Following intubation, ventilation need *not* be synchronized with chest compressions.

Indications in ACLS

Cardiac Arrest

Immediately after failure of initial attempts at defibrillation or upon determination of *asystole* or *pulseless electrical activity* (PEA), the task of intubation is assigned by the team leader.

Other Indications

- Inability of the patient to ventilate adequately or protect their airway.
- Inability of the rescuer to ventilate adequately using other methods.

Prevention of Complications

Hypoxia During Procedure

Preoxygenation and ventilation with bag–mask–oral airway are recommended by the JAMA guidelines.

The JAMA guidelines state that attempts at intubation should not exceed 30 seconds.

Trauma

Intubation should be performed only by personnel specifically trained and experienced in this technique.

Injurious technique errors include using the upper teeth as a fulcrum, and *prying* instead of lifting the handle upward.

Esophageal or Endobronchial Intubation

The guidelines state that proper tube placement is the primary end point for the endotracheal intubation technique. Confirmation of proper placement should be achieved as follows:

- The epigastrium should be auscultated with delivery of the first breath. If left upper quadrant gurgling is *not* heard and the chest wall rises and falls, the next step is to:
- Auscultate the lung fields anteriorly at both the apices and the bases.
- The guidelines also strongly encourage the use of *end-tidal* or *exhaled carbon dioxide* detection devices. These range from simple adaptor types that change color in the presence of CO_2 to complex electronic devices. However, in cardiac arrest, these methods are *not* 100% reliable. This is because carbon dioxide exchange is impaired in low cardiac output states.
- Finally, confirmation should be obtained with a chest roentgenogram.

Endotracheal Intubation Procedure

The team leader should assign two individuals to this task. One will perform the procedure while the other provides assistance. Both the patient and the equipment must be in a proper state of readiness.

Equipment Preparation

- Appropriate endotracheal tubes must be selected. ET tubes with high-volume, low-pressure cuffs are to be used and the cuff tested for leaks. A range of internal diameter tube sizes must be available. Sizes 7.0 to 8.0 mm are recommended for females, while sizes 8.0 to 9.0 mm are often chosen for males.
- The laryngoscope light should be tested.
- A *malleable stylet* should be placed in the tube with the tip recessed about one-half inch from the end of the tube.
- Finally, the tube should be lubricated with a water-soluble gel.

Preparation of the Patient

- The patient should be placed in the *sniffing position.* As Figure 3–7 illustrates, flexing the neck and extending the head will align the axes of the mouth, the pharynx, and the trachea. This "sniffing" position allows direct visualization of the larynx. If cervical spine injury is *not* suspected, a folded towel placed under the occiput often facilitates alignment.

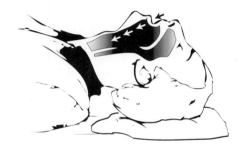

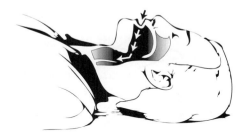

Figure 3–7. Placing the patient in the sniffing position aligns the axes of the mouth and pharynx with the axis of the trachea. A folded towel placed under the occiput often aids this process.

- At this time, the patient can be *suctioned* if necessary.
- Finally, the patient must be preoxygenated and ventilated with bag–mask ventilation.

The Intubation Procedure

The intubation procedure consists of the following four steps:

1. **Insertion of the laryngoscope blade.** As illustrated in Figure 3–8, the laryngoscope is held in the *left hand* and inserted into the right side of the mouth. The blade is then advanced gently along the natural contour of the pharynx to the base of the tongue. In so doing, the tongue is displaced to the left and the epiglottis is visualized.

2. **Visualization of the vocal cords.** Once the epiglottis is in view, it must be lifted anteriorly. This action causes the vocal cords to become visible (Figure 3–8).

    There are two types of laryngoscope blades available. Each accomplishes anterior displacement of the epiglottis in a different manner. As illustrated in Figure 3–9, when the tip of the *curved blade* is placed in the *vallecula,* upward traction results in lifting of the epiglottis. Alternatively, the *straight laryngoscope blade* may be used. This is shown in Figure 3–10.

    The straight blade is inserted *under the epiglottis.* The blade is then lifted in an upward motion. This displaces the epiglottis in such a fashion that the larynx becomes open to view.

    Proper use of either blade allows direct laryngoscopy to occur. This results in the anatomic structures of the larynx (Figure 3–8) be-

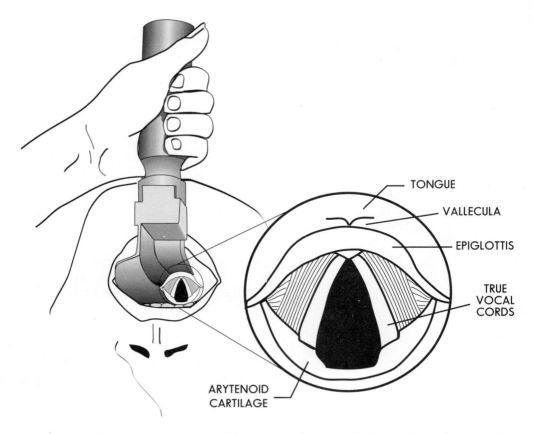

Figure 3–8. The laryngoscope is held in the left hand and advanced gently, sweeping the tongue to the left.

ing displayed. Principal among these are the pearly white folds of the vocal cords. The ET tube must be passed *between* the vocal cords until its tip is in the lower third of the trachea.

3. **Application of cricoid pressure.** The *JAMA* guidelines emphasize the importance of cricoid pressure (Sellick's maneuver) during endotracheal intubation. This procedure, which is illustrated in Figure 3–11, is performed by grasping the anterolateral aspects of the cricoid cartilage with the thumb and forefinger and applying downward pressure. This action further helps align the axes of the upper airway. It also helps protect against aspiration of gastric contents. For this reason, cricoid pressure should be maintained until the ET tube cuff is inflated.

4. **Place the endotracheal tube and inflate the cuff.** The ET tube is passed through the vocal cords. Ideally, the tip of the tube should be 2 to 4 cm from the carina. Endotracheal tubes have centimeter markings which can be used as a guide for tube placement. For adult males, markings of 21 to 23 cm at the patient's tooth line generally assures proper placement. For adult females, placing the 19 to 21 cm marks at the tooth line is usually adequate.

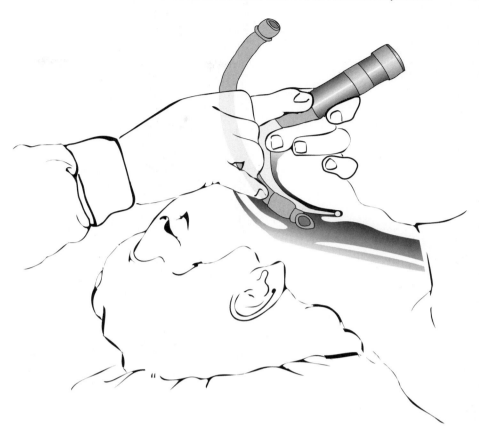

Figure 3–9. The curved blade is placed in the vallecula. This allows the epiglottis to be lifted anteriorly as upward traction is exerted.

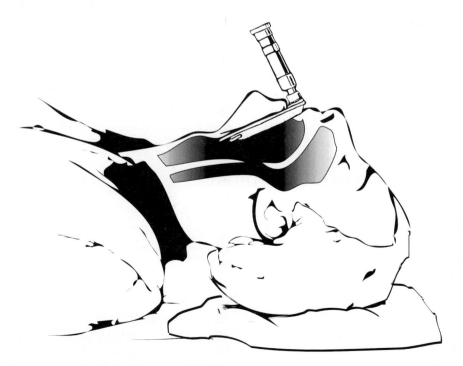

Figure 3–10. The straight blade is placed directly under the epiglottis. When the blade is lifted anteriorly, the epiglottis is displaced.

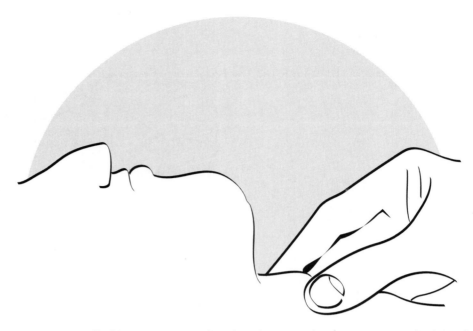

Figure 3–11. Sellick's maneuver whereby downward pressure is applied to the cricoid cartilage after being grasped between the thumb and forefinger.

Postintubation Actions

- **Ventilate and oxygenate.** Using a bag–valve unit, 100% oxygen should be delivered at a respiratory rate of 12 to 15/min using a tidal volume of 10 to 15 mL/kg. The inspiratory time should be 2 seconds.
- **Confirm tube position.** Auscultate, first over the stomach and then over both lung fields. Next, evaluate exhaled CO_2 if possible. Finally, obtain a chest x-ray as soon as possible.
- **Secure tube and chart proper "cm mark."**
- **Obtain stat arterial blood gas determination.**
- **Consider nasogastric (NG) tube placement.**

ESSENTIAL VENTILATORY ADJUNCTS

Bag–Valve Devices

Consisting of a non-rebreathing valve, a self-inflating bag, and an oxygen reservoir system, these versatile devices (Figure 3–12) can be used with endotracheal tubes, masks, or alternative airway devices. When operated using oxygen flows of 15 L/min, these units deliver F_{IO_2}s that approach 1.00.

When *bag–valve–mask* (BVM) ventilation is performed, delivery of tidal volumes in the recommended range of 10 to 15 mL/kg is facilitated by the use of an oropharyngeal airway. Two-rescuer ventilation is recom-

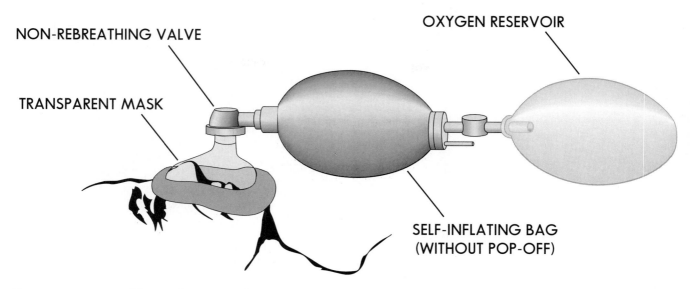

NON-REBREATHING VALVE

OXYGEN RESERVOIR

TRANSPARENT MASK

SELF-INFLATING BAG
(WITHOUT POP-OFF)

Figure 3–12. Typical bag–valve unit with oxygen reservoir system. Operated at an oxygen flow of 15 L/min, these devices deliver oxygen concentrations approaching 100%.

mended with BVM units—one to squeeze the bag and the other to ensure proper mask fit.

Standard criteria for an adult sized bag-valve unit include:

- Self-inflating and easily cleaned and sterilized.
- An oxygen inlet valve that will not jam when oxygen flows of 15 L/min are used.
- Standard 15 mm/22 mm fittings.
- An oxygen reservoir system that allows for delivery of very high oxygen concentrations.
- A true non-rebreathing valve.
- Satisfactory performance under common and extreme environmental conditions.

Pocket Mask Barrier Ventilation

Masks with a one-way valve that divert the patient's exhaled gases are a barrier ventilation method that offers the potential for the following:

- Adequate protection from cross-contamination.
- Delivery of adequate tidal volumes. Tidal volume delivery in many studies has been shown to be *superior* to BVM ventilation.
- Oxygen-enriched atmospheres can be administered. Masks equipped with oxygen inlet valves can deliver 50 to 80% oxygen at oxygen flow rates between 10 and 15 L/min (see Figure 3–13).

Face Shield Barrier Devices

Because of fear of disease transmission, health care personnel are reluctant to perform mouth-to-mouth ventilation. The Centers for Disease Control

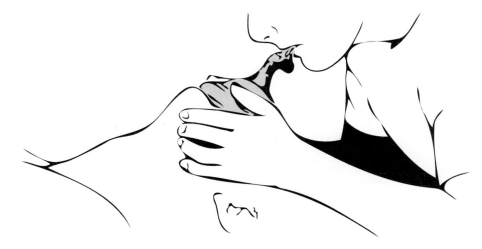

Figure 3–13. Pocket mask barrier ventilation. With the addition of an oxygen inlet valve, high concentrations of oxygen can be administered.

and Prevention (CDC) states in its guidelines that barrier devices should be used when performing rescue breathing.

In the hospital, use of barrier devices is commonplace. Bag–mask or mouth-to-mask ventilation are the initial rescue breathing methods of choice.

Face shields were developed as a barrier ventilation device for use in the pre-hospital setting. They are typically made of a flexible sheet of plastic that drapes over the face of the patient. They have a one-way ventilation valve that both provides a barrier and allows ventilation to take place. These devices have not been thoroughly studied at this time. Because of this, and the ready availability of other effective barrier devices, face shields are currently rated IIb or *possibly helpful*. Because they are disposable and easy to carry, face shield devices of acceptable design have the potential for widespread use in the pre-hospital setting.

OXYGEN ADMINISTRATION DEVICES

Nasal Cannulas

This method of oxygen administration is often preferred for the cardiac patient whose respiratory distress is mild. Recommended oxygen flow rates for this group range between 2 and 6 L/min. Since each 1 L/min via these devices is felt to increase the oxygen concentration by approximately 4%, this corresponds to oxygen concentrations of between 28 and 44%. For patients with advanced chronic obstructive pulmonary disease (COPD), 1 to 2 L/min can usually be given without fear of suppressing ventilatory drive. The JAMA guidelines stipulate, however, that oxygen should *never* be withheld for fear of this side effect and that intubation and/or assisted ventilation should always be available if needed.

Venturi Mask Devices

Another suitable method for administering oxygen to the patient with COPD is the Venturi mask. These masks employ air entrainment valves which allow for administration of precise concentrations of oxygen at high enough inspiratory flow rates that room air does not dilute the patient's inspiratory gases. Concentrations available are 24%, 28%, 35%, and 40%, with each mask being driven by 4, 4, 8, and 8 L/min of oxygen, respectively.

For the COPD patient, concentrations of 24% and 28% are usually employed initially, and the patient monitored closely for signs of ventilatory depression.

Simple Oxygen Mask

Simple oxygen masks (Figure 3–14) are well tolerated by most patients. When recommended flow rates of 8 to 10 L/min are used, these devices typically deliver oxygen concentrations between 40 and 60%.

Oxygen Masks with Reservoir

Oxygen concentrations greater than 60% are often recommended for cardiac patients who are in severe respiratory distress. These higher concentrations can be provided by either of the following types of reservoir masks.

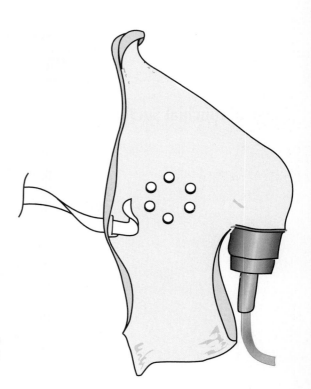

Figure 3–14. Simple oxygen masks without reservoirs provide oxygen concentrations of 40 to 60% when operated at 8 to 10 L/min.

Non-rebreathing Mask

These masks can deliver oxygen concentrations between 80 and 100% when used with flow rates of 8 to 12 L/min. Occasionally the higher flow rates may be required, as indicated by collapse of the reservoir bag during inspiration.

These devices have a one-way valve placed between the mask and the reservoir bag that prevents exhaled gases from entering the bag and thus being rebreathed. Other one-way valves are placed on the mask itself preventing entrainment of room air. In this manner, the patient theoretically inspires source gas only and his or her F_{IO_2} approaches 1.00.

Partial Rebreathing Mask

This mask is designed to deliver between 60 and 80% oxygen concentrations. This mask differs only in that the one-way valves are removed. Thus, part of the expired tidal volume enters the reservoir bag and is rebreathed. The F_{IO_2} is lowered accordingly.

SUCTIONING DEVICES AND TECHNIQUES

Pharyngeal Suctioning

During CPR and prior to endotracheal intubation, it is often necessary to clear vomitus, secretions, and other foreign material from the pharynx.

Yankauer-type rigid suctioning devices are recommended for this purpose. Proper suctioning with these devices may require negative pressures higher than 120 mm Hg.

Tracheobronchial Suctioning

During ACLS, suctioning of the trachea and of the bronchi *through the endotracheal tube* is performed with standard flexible suction catheters.

The JAMA guideline emphasize the following key points with regard to tracheobronchial suctioning:

- Suction pressures used should be between -80 and -120 mm Hg.
- The patient should be preoxygenated for 5 minutes with 100% oxygen.
- Sterile technique should be used, and suction applied *only* as the catheter is withdrawn.
- Suctioning should not be applied for more than 15 seconds.
- Before repeating the procedure, the patient should be ventilated with 100% oxygen for 30 seconds.

Complications of tracheobronchial suctioning include:

- **Hypoxemia.** This is due to interruption of ventilation and the evacuation of lung volume.
- **Arrhythmias.** Both bradyarrhythmias and tachyarrhythmias are common complications. Their presence is related respectively to vagal stimulation and hypoxemia.
- **Increased intercranial pressure.** This can result from forceful coughing.
- **Bleeding and trauma.** "Jabbing" of the catheter is to be avoided, as is the use of excessive suction pressure.

ENDOTRACHEAL DRUG ADMINISTRATION

While venous access is being established, various fat-soluble drugs can be administered via the ET tube.

Atropine, lidocaine, and epinephrine can be remembered using the mnemonic ALE. *Naloxone* and *diazepam* can also be administered by this route. The JAMA guidelines recommend the following procedure:

- 2.0 to 2.5 times the recommended IV dose should be diluted in 10 mL of either normal saline or distilled water.
- Compression should be stopped.
- If available, a long catheter should be passed beyond the tip of the ET tube.
- The solution can then be sprayed into the lungs.
- The patient should be bagged quickly several times to distribute the medication.
- Compressions should be resumed.

BIBLIOGRAPHY

1. American Heart Association, Emergency Cardiac Care Committee and Subcommittees. Guidelines for cardiopulmonary resuscitation and emergency cardiac care. JAMA 1992;268:2171–2295
2. American Heart Association. Textbook of advanced cardiac life support. Dallas, TX: American Heart Association, 1994
3. American Heart Association. Instructor's manual for advanced cardiac life support. Dallas, TX: American Heart Association, 1994
4. American Society of Anesthesiologists Task Force. Practice guidelines for management of the difficult airway. Anesthesiology 1993;78:597–602
5. Bishop Michael J. Practice guidelines for airway care during resuscitation. Respir Care 1995;40:393–403
6. Branson RD. Techniques of emergency ventilation. Respir Care 1995;40:497–497
7. Pepe PE, Zachariah BS, Chandra N. Invasive airway techniques in resuscitation. Ann Emerg Med 1993;22:(2, Part 2):393–403
8. Simmons M, Deao D, Moon L, Peters K, Cavanaugh S. Bench evaluation: Three face-shield CPR barrier devices. Respir Care 1995;40:618–623

9. Thalman JJ, Rinaldo-Gallo S, MacIntyre NR. Analysis of an endotracheal intubation service provided by respiratory care practitioners. Respir Care 1993;38(5): 469–473

10. Zyla EL, Carlson J. Respiratory care practitioners as secondary providers of endotracheal intubation: One hospital's experience. Respir Care 1994;39(1):30–33

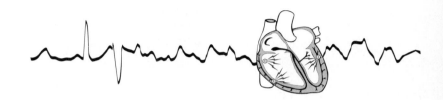

4. Defibrillation and Transcutaneous Pacemakers

OUTLINE

Essential ACLS Curricula

Definition of Terms

Importance of Early Defibrillation

Transthoracic Impedance

Electrode Size, Type, and Placement

Energy Recommendations for Defibrillation

Energy Recommendations for Cardioversion

Precordial Thump

Defibrillation in Asystole

Automated External Defibrillation

Transcutaneous Pacemakers

The Bradycardia Algorithm

ESSENTIAL ACLS CURRICULA

The American Heart Association's (AHA) *Instructor's Manual for Advanced Cardiac Life Support* has designated the following skills as necessary for completion of an essential ACLS provider course:

- Defibrillation with automated external defibrillators (AEDs)
- Defibrillation with conventional defibrillators
- Precordial thump defibrillation
- Electrical cardioversion with conventional defibrillators
- Transcutaneous pacemakers to provide both *synchronous* and *demand* pacing

The following modes of electrical therapy are considered *supplemental curricula* and are taught only in a comprehensive ACLS course. They are thus beyond the scope of this review text.

- Transvenous pacing
- Permanent pacemakers
- Automatic implantable cardioverter–defibrillator (AICD) devices

DEFINITION OF TERMS

Proper understanding of electrical therapy requires understanding of the following terms:

Countershock

This is the use of an electric shock applied to the heart to terminate an arrhythmia. Countershock is successful because it depolarizes the entire myocardium, producing a period of *asystole*. After this period of asystole, the sinus node often resumes its role as the dominant pacemaker.

Joules

The energy of the countershock is measured in joules. A joule is the number of watts of power delivered times the duration of the impulse in seconds. Thus, the unit for the electrical term *joule* is watt · second.

Defibrillation

This is the process of administering an unsynchronized countershock to terminate ventricular fibrillation (VF). Because VF is a chaotic rhythm without demonstrable R waves, the countershock cannot be delivered synchronously with an R wave. Similarly, defibrillation is often necessary when ventricular tachycardia is extremely rapid or polymorphic.

Synchronized Cardioversion

This is the technique of delivering an electrical shock to terminate arrhythmias which *do* have an R wave. These include the following:

- Ventricular tachycardia (VT)
- Atrial fibrillation
- Atrial flutter
- Paryxosymal supraventricular tachycardia (PSVT)

Conventional defibrillators have a synchronizer switch. When the defibrillator is activated and this switch is in the "on" position, the device will elec-

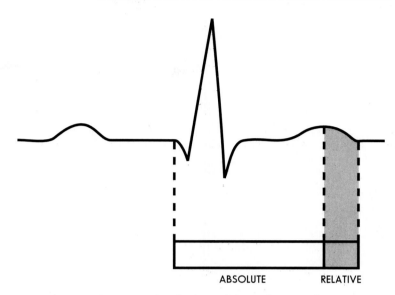

Figure 4–1. Delivery of countershock during the relative refractory period of the cardiac cycle can precipitate ventricular tachycardia or fibrillation.

tronically "hunt" for the next R wave. Upon location, it will countershock within a few milliseconds. In this way, the ACLS provider avoids precipitating ventricular fibrillation as a result of delivering an action potential during the *relative refractory period* illustrated in Figure 4–1. As will be discussed in Chapter 6, the T wave, which represents ventricular *repolarization*, is the most vulnerable portion of the heart's electrical cycle.

IMPORTANCE OF EARLY DEFIBRILLATION

The primary goal of ACLS is to provide *early* and appropriate treatment for cardiac arrest. Defibrillation is the *only* effective therapy for ventricular fibrillation and pulseless ventricular tachycardia (VF/VT). Other relevant facts include:

- 80 to 90% of all episodes of cardiac arrest are caused by VF/VT.
- When defibrillation is performed within two minutes of the onset of VF/VT, this therapy is successful roughly 80% of the time.
- When defibrillation is delayed ten minutes after the start of VF/VT, the survival rate is less than 10%.

These statistics are illustrated in Figure 4–2.

This data explains why *providing early defibrillation is the most important goal of ACLS*. Early application of CPR contributes to successful outcomes, but CPR alone cannot restore a viable rhythm.

As pictured in Figure 4–2, there is an 8-minute window of time during which survival rates soar from 10 to 80%. Mindful of this, ACLS providers have reason to be optimistic about the future. This is because the widespread use of automated external defibrillators (AEDs) promises to pare minutes from rescuer response times.

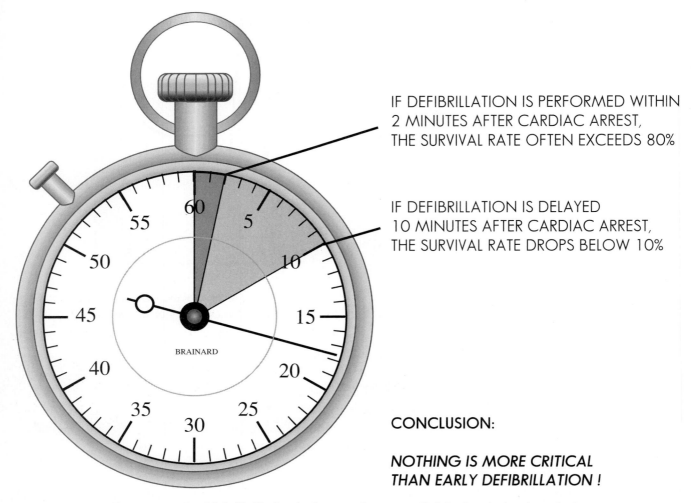

IF DEFIBRILLATION IS PERFORMED WITHIN 2 MINUTES AFTER CARDIAC ARREST, THE SURVIVAL RATE OFTEN EXCEEDS 80%

IF DEFIBRILLATION IS DELAYED 10 MINUTES AFTER CARDIAC ARREST, THE SURVIVAL RATE DROPS BELOW 10%

CONCLUSION:

NOTHING IS MORE CRITICAL THAN EARLY DEFIBRILLATION !

Figure 4–2. Rapid defibrillation is the most important link in the chain of survival.

Properly placed in homes and public places, AEDs have the potential to achieve dramatic improvements in mortality and morbidity from sudden arrhythmic death.

TRANSTHORACIC IMPEDANCE

Even if the proper level of energy is chosen, electrical conversion may be prohibited if resistance to electrical current across the thorax is excessive. Ways to minimize transthoracic impedance to countershock include:

- "Stacking" of shocks. Transthoracic impedance *decreases* with repeated shocks. Thus, even if subsequent shocks are given using the same energy, current delivery will increase.
- Firm pressure against the chest wall when using handheld paddle electrodes.
- Use of conductive gel or pads between paddles and skin.

- Use of large (8 to 12 cm) adhesive chest wall electrodes will also provide minimal chest wall impedance despite the fact that "paddle pressure" is not employed.

ELECTRODE SIZE, TYPE, AND PLACEMENT

Size of Electrode

For both hand-held paddle-type and self-adhesive electrodes, diameters of 8 to 12 cm are recommended.

Type of Electrode

Conventional defibrillators use hand-held paddles which allow the user to lower transthoracic impedance by bearing down firmly as countershock is being administered. Modern self-adhesive electrodes, because of their large surface-to-skin contact area, are felt to provide equally low resistance to current flow.

Defibrillators that allow remote delivery of countershock through cables to these efficient self-adhesive electrodes are valuable because they enhance operator safety. It is not difficult to appreciate the advantage of being able to perform remote defibrillation in a cramped ambulance or helicopter.

Electrode Placement

Figure 4–3 illustrates the *anterior–apex* or *sternal–apex* electrode position commonly used in providing defibrillation. In this position, one electrode is placed to the right of the sternum, below the clavicle and the other

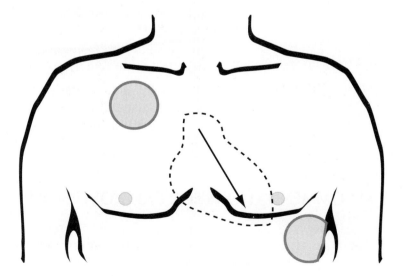

Figure 4–3. The anterior–apex position traditionally used for defibrillation attempts.

is positioned to the left of the nipple, with the electrode in the midaxillary line.

An alternative placement position is to place one electrode directly over the left precordium and the other directly behind it in the right infrascapular location. This *anterior–posterior* placement scheme is often employed when using newer generation defibrillators that have transcutaneous pacing (TCP) capabilities. These units feature multifunctional electrodes that can be used for remote countershock, transcutaneous pacing (TCP), and ECG monitoring.

ENERGY RECOMMENDATIONS FOR DEFIBRILLATION

As illustrated in the VF/pulseless VT algorithm (Figure 4–4), defibrillation, if indicated, is accomplished as soon as a defibrillator can be attached. CPR is to be performed until then. You will note that defibrillation is administered up to three times in a row to treat VF/VT.

The *JAMA* guidelines recommend that these three unsynchronized shocks be delivered in a *stacked* manner, with only enough time taken in between to recharge the defibrillator and to confirm the presence or absence of VF/VT.

During this time, as electrodes remain on the chest, the team leader must remind all personnel to *stay clear* of the bed and the patient. This means that CPR is *not* to be performed at this time. The energy sequence recommended by the guidelines is:

- 200 joules for the first shock
- 200 to 300 joules for the second shock
- 360 joules for the third shock

If these three stacked electrical shocks fail to convert VF/VT to a viable rhythm, the following steps should be ordered by the team leader:

- Resumption of CPR
- Intubation of the trachea
- IV access
- Administration of epinephrine by first route available (the initial IV dose is 1.0 mg of a 1:10,000 solution).

If VF/VT persists, defibrillation is performed once again at 360 joules. Finally, medications rated IIa (probably helpful) in the algorithm are to be alternated with defibrillation at 360 J. The pattern should be *drug–shock, drug–shock.*

ENERGY RECOMMENDATIONS FOR CARDIOVERSION

The purpose of synchronized cardioversion is to prevent delivery of electrical energy during the *relative refractory period* of the heart's electrical cycle.

Ventricular Fibrillation/Pulseless Ventricular Tachycardia (VF/VT) Algorithm

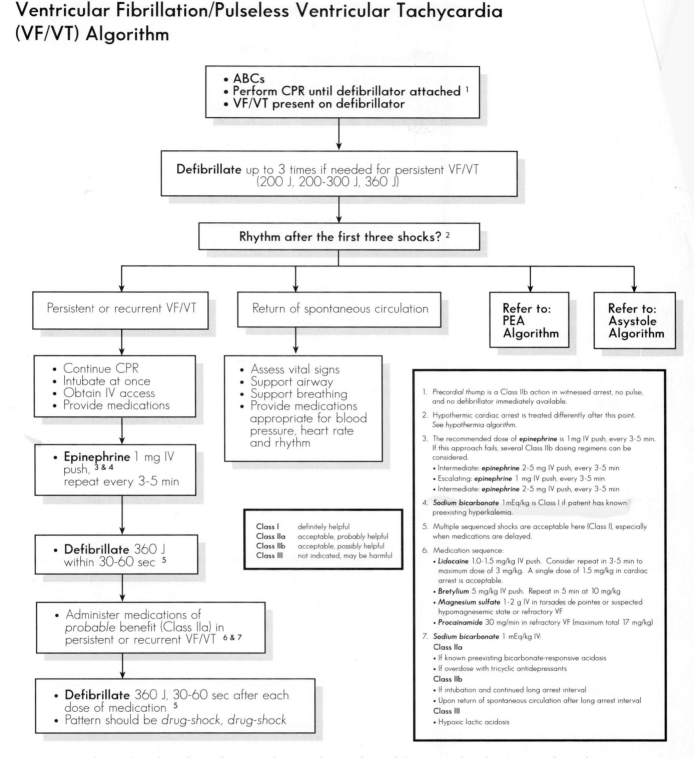

Figure 4–4. The VF/VT algorithm. The provider's understanding of this critical pathway is evaluated in Case 3, Mega VF–Refractory VF/VT. (Algorithm copyright 1992, American Medical Association; JAMA, October 28, 1992; pp 2199–2241.)

As illustrated in the electrical cardioversion algorithm (Figure 4–5), synchronized countershock is indicated in the treatment of excessively rapid and/or hemodynamically unstable tachycardias of both *ventricular* and *supraventricular* origin. You will note that the algorithm contains the following protocols for these arrhythmias:

- Ventricular tachycardia and atrial fibrillation: 100 J, 200 J, 300 J, 360 J
- Atrial flutter and PSVT: 50 J, 100 J, 200 J, 300 J, 360 J

Please appreciate that sinus tachycardia does not appear on this list. The reason is that the purpose of electrical countershock is to *induce* a sinus

Electrical Cardioversion/Unstable Tachycardia Algorithm
(Patient not in cardiac arrest)

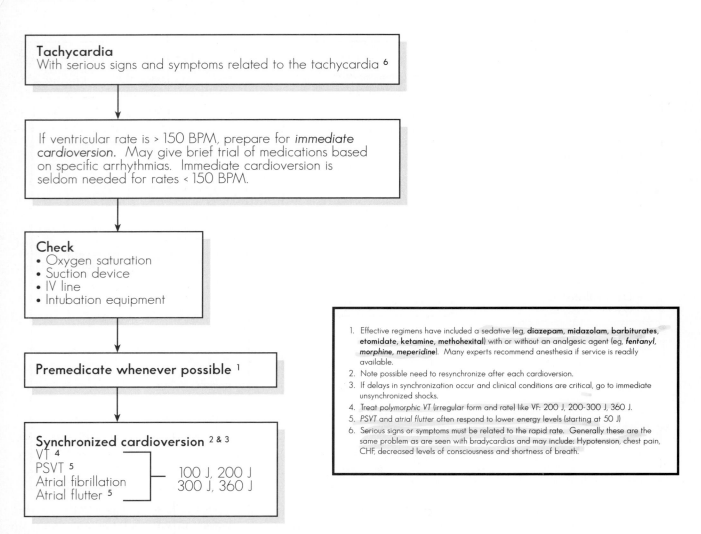

Tachycardia
With serious signs and symptoms related to the tachycardia [6]

If ventricular rate is > 150 BPM, prepare for *immediate cardioversion*. May give brief trial of medications based on specific arrhythmias. Immediate cardioversion is seldom needed for rates < 150 BPM.

Check
- Oxygen saturation
- Suction device
- IV line
- Intubation equipment

Premedicate whenever possible [1]

Synchronized cardioversion [2 & 3]
VT [4]
PSVT [5]
Atrial fibrillation
Atrial flutter [5]
— 100 J, 200 J 300 J, 360 J

1. Effective regimens have included a sedative (eg, **diazepam, midazolam, barbiturates, etomidate, ketamine, methohexital**) with or without an analgesic agent (eg, **fentanyl, morphine, meperidine**). Many experts recommend anesthesia if service is readily available.
2. Note possible need to resynchronize after each cardioversion.
3. If delays in synchronization occur and clinical conditions are critical, go to immediate unsynchronized shocks.
4. Treat polymorphic VT (irregular form and rate) like VF: 200 J, 200-300 J, 360 J.
5. *PSVT* and *atrial flutter* often respond to lower energy levels (starting at 50 J)
6. Serious signs or symptoms must be related to the rapid rate. Generally these are the same problem as are seen with bradycardias and may include: Hypotension, chest pain, CHF, decreased levels of consciousness and shortness of breath.

Figure 4–5. Electrical cardioversion algorithm for unstable tachycardia. Understanding of this critical pathway is evaluated in Case 8, Unstable Tachycardia/Electrical Cardioversion. (Algorithm copyright 1992, American Medical Association; JAMA, October 28, 1992; pp 2199–2241.)

rhythm. Also note that these arrhythmias require synchronized counter-shock because, unlike ventricular fibrillation, they have an R wave. That said, it must be added that when ventricular tachycardia is polymorphic or rapid delays in synchronization are common. In this case, the operator must proceed *immediately* with defibrillation.

The procedure for providing synchronized cardioversion is presented in Figure 4–5. This critical pathway directs that synchronized cardioversion be administered immediately if an *unstable tachycardia* exists. The guidelines define an unstable tachycardia as follows:

- Ventricular rate greater than 150/min with serious signs and symptoms *related to the tachycardia.*
- Serious *symptoms* include shortness of breath, chest pain, and decreased levels of consciousness.
- Serious *signs* include systolic BP less than 80 mm Hg, poor perfusion, jugular venous distention, and congestive heart failure (CHF).

The algorithm states that rates less than 150/min are *seldom* unstable enough to require immediate cardioversion. The JAMA guidelines, however, issue a cautionary refrain to "treat the patient, not the monitor."

The next steps in this algorithm involve ensuring patient comfort and safety. Thus, the provider is instructed to assess and assure the following:

- Oxygen saturation levels
- Proper operation of suctioning equipment
- IV line
- Intubation equipment
- Premedication of the patient wherever possible

Finally, after all necessary preparations have been made, the provider should select the energy sequence specified in the algorithm.

PRECORDIAL THUMP

The precordial thump is a potentially hazardous procedure that is not taught as part of BCLS.

An ACLS technique only, the JAMA guidelines give it a IIb (possibly helpful) classification for optional use in a witnessed cardiac arrest where the patient is pulseless and where a defibrillator is not immediately available.

The thump is delivered as a single sharp blow to the center of the sternum from a height of no more than 12 inches, using the ulnar aspect of the clenched fist. This delivers a low-energy shock of approximately 4 joules to the myocardium. This has been shown to *occasionally* convert VF/VT of recent onset.

DEFIBRILLATION IN ASYSTOLE

Studies have not revealed any benefit or improvement in outcomes resulting from the use of defibrillation to treat asystole. For this reason, it is *not* a part of the asystole treatment algorithm presented in the JAMA guidelines.

The guidelines, however, are quick to emphasize that when the ACLS provider confronts an isoelectric line on the monitor, he or she must quickly rule out *false asystole*. Typically, this is the result of one of the following two scenarios:

Operator Error!

Operator error is the most common cause of false asystole. Rapid attention must be paid to the following:

- Loose leads
- No power
- Disconnection of lead lines

Isoelectric VF

Less frequently, VF/VT may resemble asystole in an isolated lead. Therefore, asystole must be *confirmed* by observing its presence in *several* leads.

AUTOMATED EXTERNAL DEFIBRILLATION

The Need for AEDs

Early defibrillation is the most important link in the chain of survival. The guidelines estimate that survival from ventricular fibrillation drops 7 to 10% for each minute that defibrillation is delayed following cardiac arrest.

Automated external defibrillators (AEDs) (Figure 4–6) offer the potential to cut minutes off the delivery time associated with conventional defibrillators. Additionally, AED devices require little training for proper use. Because of these vital reasons, AEDs are being placed throughout the community as rapidly as resources allow.

Types of AEDs

An AED is an external defibrillator that can electronically determine the presence or absence of ventricular fibrillation. There are two types of AEDs. Both have been extensively tested and are considered equally safe.

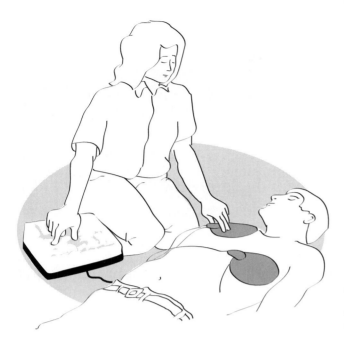

Figure 4–6. The automated external defibrillator (AED). These devices are seeing widespread use in the community at large. Proper use can be taught during a basic CPR course. A computer chip does most of the work.

Fully Automated AEDs

These are often preferred for use by operators with modest training, such as family members and non-public safety personnel. Operation is simple, consisting of the following three actions:

- Determine *unconsciousness* and *pulselessness*
- Attach defibrillator pads
- Activate "on" control

Shock Advisory AEDs

Shock advisory AEDs, as illustrated in Figure 4–7, require two additional steps to accomplish defibrillation. Because they are not left out of the decision-making process, these devices are preferred by trained health care personnel. Their operational procedure is as follows:

- Determine *unconsciousness* and *pulselessness*
- Attach defibrillator pads
- Activate "on" control
- Activate *analysis* mode

Unlike fully automated AEDs, these devices will *not* perform rhythm evaluation until the analysis mode is selected.

- Activate defibrillation or "shock" control

Once the device has performed its analysis, it will then "advise" the operator of the presence or absence of a *shockable rhythm.*

Should VF be detected, the operator must then press the "shock" control each time he or she is required to perform defibrillation.

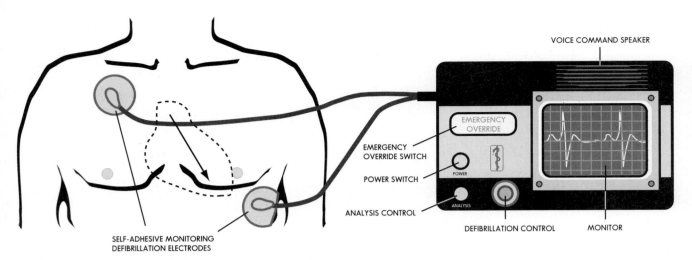

Figure 4–7. The shock advisory-type AED. These compact automated devices make it possible for persons with minimal training to deliver life-saving defibrillation. A computer chip does most of the work. The operator must: (1) determine pulselessness and unconsciousness; (2) attach electrodes; (3) press "analyze" button; and (4) press "defibrillation" button, if so commanded.

Comparison of Automated and Conventional Defibrillatory Techniques

With conventional defibrillation, rhythm analysis is performed by a trained individual. With automated defibrillation, this function is performed electronically. The JAMA guidelines compare the two methods as follows.

Accuracy of Rhythm Analysis

The guidelines state that the rhythm detection ability of AEDs is comparable to that of pre-hospital emergency personnel, trained to administer conventional defibrillation. Episodes of faulty rhythm analysis and inappropriate shock delivery are rare and are usually related to one of the following situations:

- **Motion artifact.** AED devices are somewhat of a technological miracle in that they are seldom led astray by patient muscular or respiratory artifact. Unfortunately, this is *not* the case with transport artifact. Thus, AEDs must only be placed in the analysis mode when the ambulance is at a complete stop. *Additionally, CPR must not be performed while analysis is being performed.*
- **Failure to recognize rare varieties of VF or VT.** Occasionally, AEDs may fail to shock extremely fine or coarse varieties of ventricular fibrillation. Remarkably, these devices will shock both monomorphic and polymorphic ventricular tachycardia if the rate exceeds threshold values.

Speed of Delivery

In a benchmark comparison, clinical trials report delivery of the first shock an average of 1 minute sooner than emergency personnel using conventional defibrillation. Critical delivery time is expected to improve as more AEDs are placed throughout the community.

Training Required for Proper Operation

Learning to operate AED devices is felt to require less training than basic CPR. Necessary skills are:

- Ability to recognize unconsciousness and pulselessness
- Ability to attach defibrillator pads properly
- Ability to learn AED algorithm (Figure 4–8)

The AED Critical Pathway

The AED treatment pathway illustrated in Figure 4–8 outlines the steps to be used in treating the patient with cardiac arrest, using an AED device.

Step I: Determine Need for Defibrillation

Immediately after determining the presence of pulselessness, rescuers should begin performing CPR. Simultaneously, an additional rescuer should attach the AED's electrode pads to the patient in a modified lead II position. The AED is subsequently turned on and placed in the *analysis* mode.

It is imperative to note that the patient must *not* be touched while the AED analyzes the rhythm. *This means that CPR efforts must cease.* Only in this way can chances of inappropriate shocks to the victim and to rescuers be minimized.

Rhythm assessment and capacitor charging usually takes 5 to 15 seconds. If VF/VT is present, the AED's command system will announce that a shock is needed.

Step II: Defibrillate Times Three if Commanded (200 J, 200–300 J, 360 J)

To prevent injury, the operator must first make sure that everyone is *clear* of the patient! This is done immediately after the shock command is issued *before* the shock control is activated.

The three shocks must be "stacked." Thus, after each shock, the only action taken is to press the ANALYZE control.

Pulse checks are *not* to be performed until after the third shock, unless the "no shock indicated" command is issued.

Automated External Defibrillation (AED) Critical Pathway*

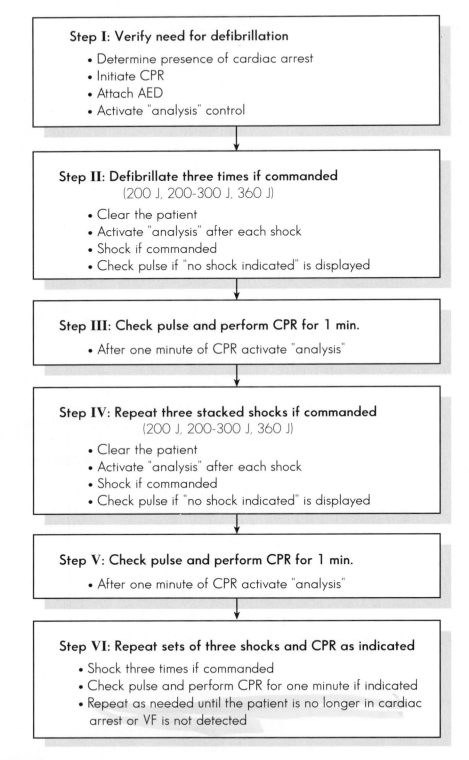

Step I: Verify need for defibrillation

- Determine presence of cardiac arrest
- Initiate CPR
- Attach AED
- Activate "analysis" control

Step II: Defibrillate three times if commanded
(200 J, 200-300 J, 360 J)

- Clear the patient
- Activate "analysis" after each shock
- Shock if commanded
- Check pulse if "no shock indicated" is displayed

Step III: Check pulse and perform CPR for 1 min.

- After one minute of CPR activate "analysis"

Step IV: Repeat three stacked shocks if commanded
(200 J, 200-300 J, 360 J)

- Clear the patient
- Activate "analysis" after each shock
- Shock if commanded
- Check pulse if "no shock indicated" is displayed

Step V: Check pulse and perform CPR for 1 min.

- After one minute of CPR activate "analysis"

Step VI: Repeat sets of three shocks and CPR as indicated

- Shock three times if commanded
- Check pulse and perform CPR for one minute if indicated
- Repeat as needed until the patient is no longer in cardiac arrest or VF is not detected

Figure 4–8. The AED Critical Pathway. Understanding of this critical pathway is evaluated in Case 2: Witnessed Adult Cardiac Arrest. *Please refer to the AED treatment algorithm in your AHA textbook of ACLS for additional information.

AEDs are programmed to select the proper level of power for each indicated shock.

Step III: Check Pulse and Perform CPR

As the AED algorithm indicates, if the victim is still pulseless, CPR is to be performed for one minute. If after this time the victim remains pulseless, the operator must once again activate the ANALYZE control.

If VF/VT is still present, the AED will issue the appropriate command, causing the operator to:

Step IV: Repeat Three "Stacked" Shocks at up to 360 Joules

Once again, the only action to be taken in between shocks is to activate the ANALYSIS control. After the third stacked shock, the operator is instructed to perform a pulse check and administer CPR for one minute if it is absent. If after this the victim is still without a pulse, the rescuer must:

Step V: Repeat the Sequence of Three "Stacked" Shocks

Finally, the algorithm stipulates that sets of three stacked shocks, followed by one minute of CPR, be repeated until a perfusing rhythm is achieved.

TRANSCUTANEOUS PACEMAKERS

Advantages Over Transvenous Pacemakers in ACLS

In consideration of the fact that JAMA guidelines deal with the emergency cardiac care of the AMI patient, it is not suprising that the role they describe for invasive procedures such as transvenous pacemakers is a supplemental one.

There are a number of reasons why transcutaneous pacemakers are the preferred method in ACLS. Largely practical considerations, these include:

Safety

Administered without the need for vascular access, it is the most suitable means of providing pacing for patients who have or may require thrombolytic therapy. In addition, the modern transcutaneous pacemaker is able to achieve capture at much lower levels of current than earlier models. Thus, risks such as induction of VF, burns to the victim, and electrical shock to operators, have virtually been eliminated.

Widespread Availability

Most defibrillators currently manufactured offer a built-in transcutaneous pacemaker. Through a single pair of adhesive electrodes, the operator has the choice of remote pacing, ECG monitoring, and defibrillation.

Anterior–posterior chest wall electrode placement is employed when external pacing is desired, although *anterior–apex* positioning is considered an acceptable alternative.

Ease of Operation

The modern transcutaneous pacemaker is easily applied and operated. Training requirements are not considered excessive. Thus, these devices can be used by a wide variety of non-physician personnel in both pre-hospital and acute care settings.

The Technique of Transcutaneous Pacing

Transcutaneous pacemakers (TCPs) are capable of operating in both a *fixed* (asynchronous) and a *demand* (synchronous) mode. Typically, the demand mode is used because it greatly reduces the chances of precipitating ventricular fibrillation. This can result when pacing potentials are delivered during the *relative refractory period* of the electrical cycle (see Figure 4–1).

Most TCPs allow a range of rates from 30 to 180 beats per minute to be selected. Current output is generally adjustable from 0 to 200 mA. Most patients require between 50 and 100 mA to achieve capture. The technique for transcutaneous pacing is as follows.

Attach Electrodes

Anterior–posterior electrode placement is preferred. However, anterior–apex positioning is acceptable (see Figure 4–3).

Activate the Device

Starting with a rate of 80/min is usually acceptable.

Adjust Current Levels to Achieve Capture

In patients who are pulseless, it may be wise to employ initial current settings of 150 to 200 mA and then decrease these levels once capture is achieved. In patients who are symptomatic, yet conscious, it is advisable to apply current incrementally.

Electrical capture is determined by ECG analysis, using the monitor on the pacemaker device itself. These monitors employ special filters that electronically "blank" out pacemaker spike-induced artifact.

As can be seen in Figure 4–9, electrical capture is normally accompanied by widening of the QRS complex and the presence of a broad T wave.

In Figure 4–9, the broad pacemaker spike that is characteristic of transcutaneous pacing can also be seen.

Precautions with Transcutaneous Pacemakers

- **Pain and discomfort.** Most conscious patients will experience a considerable degree of discomfort from this procedure. In light of this, the guidelines recommend that appropriate analgesia and sedation be employed.

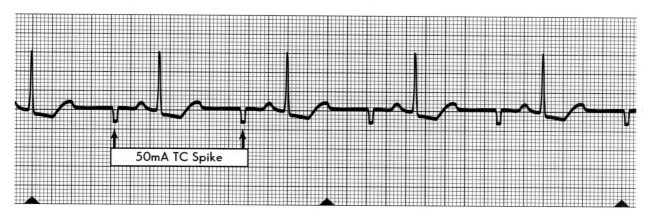

A. Patient with sinus bradycardia (rate 42/min.) and failure to capture. Note that electronically filtered TCP impulses are morphologically different from transvenous pacer spikes.

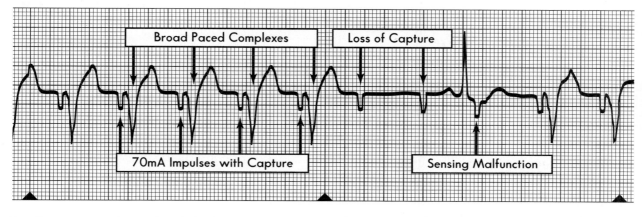

B. Capture is achieved with higher current pacing impulse (70mA). Note that the paced QRS complexes and their T-waves are characteristically broad.

Figure 4–9. In these illustrations, capture is achieved with 70-mA pacing impulse but is lost temporarily. A slightly higher current level should be employed in this case so capture can be held. When a pacing impulse is delivered during the refractory part of the electrical cycle, it is termed a sensing malfunction.

- **Failure to achieve capture.** This has been reported in patients who are barrel chested and in those who have pericardial fluid. The presence of intrathoracic air and fluid can greatly increase the energy required for capture.
- **Failure to recognize underlying treatable VF.** This has been documented and is usually related to the use of older ECG monitors that lack "blanking" circuitry. Nonfiltered pacemaker-induced artifact can mask lethal arrhythmias. Even when modern devices are used operators must always monitor the ECG carefully as large pacer spikes can present a confusing picture.

THE BRADYCARDIA ALGORITHM

The bradycardia algorithm (Figure 4–10) outlines the ACLS management of patients who are bradycardic. These patients must initially be evaluated to determine the presence of serious signs and symptoms related to the slow rhythm. These signs and symptoms are the same ones that are used to assess unstable tachycardia (see Figure 4–5).

Serious *symptoms* include chest pain, shortness of breath, and obtundation. Serious *signs* include systolic BP less than 80 mm Hg, poor perfusion, jugular venous distention, and CHF.

The JAMA guidelines strongly suggest that the seriousness of the clinical situation be confirmed by the presence of more than one of these deleterious markers.

The bradycardia algorithm specifies two class I (definitely helpful) indications for TCP use in ACLS. These are discussed below.

Second-degree Type II AV Block and Third-degree AV Block

These two serious arrhythmias are associated with acute anterior MI and infranodal block at the Purkinje level. These patients typically rely on an ideoventricular escape pacemaker and usually have an unstable clinical status. When this is the case, a transcutaneous pacemaker should be placed immediately while the patient is prepared for insertion of a *transvenous* pacemaker.

Standby pacing with a TCP device is indicated for hemodynamically stable patients who present with these arrhythmias. In this instance, mechanical capture and patient tolerance should be verified on a trial basis. Decompensation must be anticipated and the patient monitored accordingly.

Symptomatic Bradycardias

Transcutaneous pacing is a class I intervention in *all* symptomatic bradycardias. It should be initiated promptly in bradycardic patients who have suffered an AMI, those who are symptomatic, *and* those who do not respond promptly to atropine.

Bradycardia Algorithm
(Patient is not in cardiac arrest)

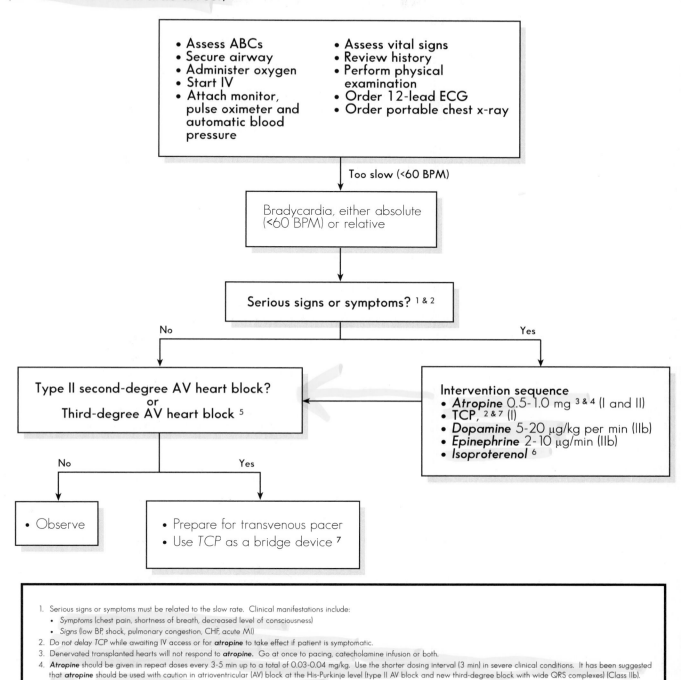

Assess ABCs
- Secure airway
- Administer oxygen
- Start IV
- Attach monitor, pulse oximeter and automatic blood pressure

- Assess vital signs
- Review history
- Perform physical examination
- Order 12-lead ECG
- Order portable chest x-ray

Too slow (<60 BPM)

Bradycardia, either absolute (<60 BPM) or relative

Serious signs or symptoms? [1 & 2]

No

Yes

Type II second-degree AV heart block?
or
Third-degree AV heart block [5]

Intervention sequence
- *Atropine* 0.5-1.0 mg [3 & 4] (I and II)
- *TCP*, [2 & 7] (I)
- *Dopamine* 5-20 µg/kg per min (IIb)
- *Epinephrine* 2-10 µg/min (IIb)
- *Isoproterenol* [6]

No

Yes

- Observe

- Prepare for transvenous pacer
- Use *TCP* as a bridge device [7]

1. Serious signs or symptoms must be related to the slow rate. Clinical manifestations include:
   - Symptoms (chest pain, shortness of breath, decreased level of consciousness)
   - Signs (low BP, shock, pulmonary congestion, CHF, acute MI)
2. Do not delay TCP while awaiting IV access or for **atropine** to take effect if patient is symptomatic.
3. Denervated transplanted hearts will not respond to **atropine**. Go at once to pacing, catecholamine infusion or both.
4. **Atropine** should be given in repeat doses every 3-5 min up to a total of 0.03-0.04 mg/kg. Use the shorter dosing interval (3 min) in severe clinical conditions. It has been suggested that **atropine** should be used with caution in atrioventricular (AV) block at the His-Purkinje level (type II AV block and new third-degree block with wide QRS complexes) (Class IIb).
5. Never treat third-degree heart block plus ventricular escape beats with **lidocaine.**
6. **Isoproterenol** should be used, if at all, with extreme caution. At low doses it is a Class IIb (possibly helpful). At higher doses it is a Class III (harmful).
7. Verify patient tolerance and mechanical capture. Use analgesia and sedation as needed.

Figure 4–10. The bradycardia algorithm. The provider's understanding of this critical pathway is assessed in Case 7, Bradycardia. (Algorithm copyright 1992, American Medical Association; JAMA, October 28, 1992; pp 2199–2241.)

Hypotensive and bradycardic patients who do not respond to atropine should receive an intravenous infusion of *dopamine* or *epinephrine* until capture can be achieved.

BIBLIOGRAPHY

1. American Heart Association. Emergency Cardiac Care Committee and Subcommittees. Guidelines for cardiopulmonary resuscitation and emergency cardiac care. JAMA 1992;268:2171–2295
2. American Heart Association. Textbook of advanced cardiac life support. Dallas, TX: American Heart Association, 1994
3. American Heart Association. Instructor's manual for advanced cardiac life support. Dallas, TX: American Heart Association, 1994
4. Aufderheide T. Pacemakers and electrical therapy during advanced cardiac life support. Respir Care 1995;40(4):364–379
5. Cummins RO, Ornato JP, Thies WH, Pepe PE. Improving survival from sudden cardiac death: the "chain of survival" concept. Circulation 1991;83:1832–1847
6. Cummins RO, Theis W, Paraskos J, Kerber RE, Billi JE, Seidel J, et al. Encouraging early defibrillation: the American Heart Association and automated external defibrillators. Ann Emerg Med 1990;19:1245–1248
7. Hargarten KM, Stueven HA, Waite EM, Olson DW, Mateer JR, Aufderheide TP, Darin JC. Prehospital experience with defibrillation of coarse ventricular fibrillation: a ten-year review. Ann Emerg Med 1990;19:157–162
8. Watts DD: Defibrillation by basic emergency medical technicians: effect on survival. Ann Emerg Med 1995;26:635–639

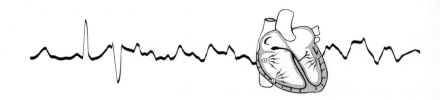

5. Intravenous Techniques

OUTLINE

ESSENTIAL ACLS CURRICULA

The *JAMA* guidelines state that unless central venous access has been established *prior* to cardiac arrest, peripheral veins are to be chosen. Because access can usually be achieved without interrupting CPR, the veins of the *antecubital fossa* or the *external jugular veins* are chosen first.

In light of this, the AHA's *Instructor's Manual for ACLS* makes the following curricular recommendations.

Essential Curricula

- Role of IV access in ACLS
- Advantages and disadvantages of peripheral vs. central IV lines
- Advantages and disadvantages of the following peripheral sites
  Antecubital
  External jugular

Dorsum of hand
Femoral
Saphenous

Supplemental Curricula for Comprehensive Courses

- Central IV lines:
  Internal jugular
  Subclavian
- Pericardiocentesis for cardiac tamponade
- Thoracentesis for pneumothorax

ROLE OF IV ACCESS DURING ACLS

The JAMA guidelines emphasize that establishment of intravenous access is a routine part of ACLS and should be accomplished as soon as possible. At the same time, they leave no doubt that during cardiac arrest, IV medications play a *secondary* role to more fundamental techniques. CPR, defibrillation, and airway care are stated to be the provider's primary focus.

Intubation of the trachea allows not only the potential to control acid–base balance, but permits administration of the following drugs.

- Oxygen
- Epinephrine
- Lidocaine
- Atropine

PRACTICAL CONSIDERATIONS IN ACLS

Indications for IV Access in ACLS

- Administration of medications
- Volume expansion
- Access to venous blood for laboratory analysis
- Central vascular catheterization

Type of Fluid and Infusion Rate

The JAMA guidelines discourage the use of 5% dextrose and other glucose-containing fluids during resuscitation. *Normal saline* or *lactated Ringer's* solutions are the preferred solutions for perfusion during ACLS.

The JAMA guidelines also recommend the use of unbreakable solution containers. When IV lines are not to be used for volume expansion, they can be kept open by setting the rate of infusion at 10 mL/h.

Hazards in ACLS

There are many hazards associated with providing IV access during ACLS. Please consider them and their relationship to central vascular infusion techniques.

Bleeding and Hematoma

Always a possible complication, it is most closely related to:

- Inexperienced operators.
- Use of subclavian, internal jugular, and femoral sites. These are not only adjacent to arteries, but can be difficult to compress.
- Administration of thrombolytic agents. Use of large (14-gauge) needles and noncompressible sites add risk when these agents are used. The JAMA guidelines state that even one unsuccessful central line attempt is a strong relative contradiction to thrombolytic therapy.

Cellulitis and Sepsis

The incidence of these complications corresponds to the fact that strict aseptic technique is not always possible during ACLS.

Phlebitis

This complication is related to cannulation of the saphenous vein *and* to the administration of hypertonic solutions through smaller peripheral veins.

Air Embolism

This is a relatively uncommon complication of internal jugular and subclavian techniques. Patients who are short of breath can generate negative pressures large enough to draw air into the venous circulation. Circulating quantities of gas can produce cardiac arrest should right ventricular contractions break these volumes into a foam.

Pneumothorax

In addition to being proximal to subclavian arteries, the subclavian veins lie close to the cupula or dome of the pleura.

Pulmonary Thromboembolism

Thrombus formation on the tip of central vascular lines is not uncommon in the acidotic or otherwise hypercoagulable patient.

Catheter Fragment Embolism

This complication is associated with the use of *catheter-through-needle systems*. If these units are used, the operator must use extreme care not to *retract* the catheter during placement. This can cause the sharp needle tip to cut the catheter in half. The catheter fragment will then become an embolus and lodge in the right heart or a pulmonary artery.

ROLE OF CENTRAL AND PERIPHERAL LINES IN ACLS

Advantages and Disadvantages of Central Lines

The JAMA guidelines state that if a central line is in place when cardiac arrest occurs, drugs should be administered via that route during ACLS.

The *advantages* offered by central infusions are worthy of consideration. Drugs so administered reach the major organs much more rapidly than when administered peripherally. In addition, these vessels are larger and less likely to collapse when poor perfusion exists.

The *disadvantages* of central sites are striking. First of all, their cannulation requires interruption of CPR. Second, while considered of low risk when performed by experienced personnel, the majority of the complications of IV techniques described above are associated with these procedures.

Advantages and Disadvantages of Peripheral Lines

Following arrest, the guidelines state that *antecubital* (see Figure 4–1) or *external jugular veins* (see Figure 4–2) are *sites of first choice*. The most important reason for this recommendation is the fact that access does not require interruption of chest compressions. Of these two sites, the external jugular veins are *least* accessible, as access is hindered by airway maintenance techniques.

Other *advantages* offered by these sites include the fact that cannulation requires less training and is associated with fewer complications than central venous techniques. In addition, these veins are relatively large and do not collapse easily. In this regard, it is worthwhile to note that during low flow states, location of the antecubital veins can be enhanced by their being draped over the side of the gurney prior to tourniquet application. In this way, the force of gravity can be employed to augment perfusion.

Their striking *disadvantage* is that drugs require 1 to 2 minutes to reach their site of action when administered via these veins. Thus, to speed the delivery of IV medications to the central circulation, the JAMA guidelines recommend that the following measures be taken:

- With few exceptions, agents should be administered rapidly, in bolus method.
- A 20-mL bolus of normal saline should be given immediately thereafter.
- Finally, the extremity should be elevated.

SELECTION OF CATHETER TYPE IN ACLS

Butterfly Type

Single hollow needles such as butterfly units are *not* recommended for use during ACLS. Reasons for this include:

- They are rigid and thus easily dislodged.
- They are too short for most applications.

Catheter *Over* Needle Units

Flexible plastic catheters which have introducer needles inside them are *recommended* for cannulation of most *peripheral* venous sites. The JAMA guidelines specify large 14- to 16-gauge cannulas because rapid volume infusion is possible if desired. Smaller (18-gauge) devices are suggested if thrombolytic agents are anticipated. Advantages offered by these units include:

- Not easily dislodged. Once the introducing core is removed, these catheters are flexible and allow unavoidable patient movement.
- They are about 5 cm long. This will allow cannulation of all but the femoral vein.
- The puncture in the vein wall is exactly the size of the cannula. This will minimize bleeding.

Catheter or *Seldinger Guidewire* Through Needle Devices

Used when *central vascular access* is required, both of these techniques require a catheter *or* a guidewire be passed *through* a needle in order to establish access. The advantage of these devices is that very long cannulas (20 cm or greater) can be introduced.

A hazard of the catheter-through-needle technique is the risk of *catheter fragment embolism*. Because it eliminates this complication, the Seldinger *guidewire*-through-needle technique is preferable.

With this procedure, a guidewire is passed through the needle into the vein. The needle is then removed. Next, the catheter is slipped *over the guidewire* and passed into the vena cavae. Finally, the guidewire is removed. This process eliminates the possibility of catheter fragment embolism.

KEY POINTS REGARDING PERIPHERAL VEIN SITES

The Antecubital Veins

As noted in Figure 5–1, important superficial veins are present on the medial aspect of the antecubital fossa. Advantages of these veins following cardiac arrest include:

- CPR does not have to be interrupted to achieve access.
- The veins are superficial and reasonably large.
- The extremity can be lowered to enhance venous filling.
- The extremity is easily elevated following agent administration. This reduces the time required for drugs to reach the central circulation.

The External Jugular Vein

Traversing the lateral portion of the neck from the middle of the clavicle to the angle of the jaw, the external jugular vein (Figure 5–2) is a recommended site following cardiac arrest. Considerations regarding this site include:

- It is much closer to the central circulation than the antecubital veins.
- Access may interrupt endotracheal intubation and airway maintenance techniques.
- It is superficial and generally easy to locate.

The Dorsal Hand Veins

The distal veins on the dorsum of the hand (Figure 5–3) are small in comparison with those in the antecubital space. The fact that this site is accessible during CPR does *not* outweigh size-related disadvantages listed below:

- Among the first to collapse during cardiac arrest.
- Size predisposes to *phlebitis.*
- Cannulas are more easily dislodged from these small veins.

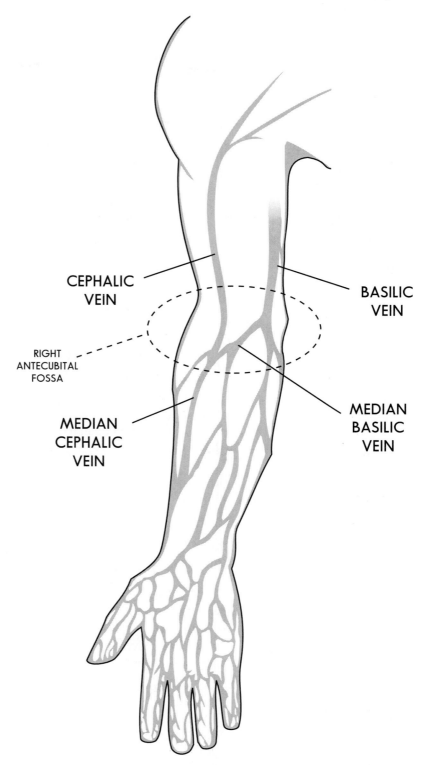

CEPHALIC
VEIN

BASILIC
VEIN

RIGHT
ANTECUBITAL
FOSSA

MEDIAN
BASILIC
VEIN

MEDIAN
CEPHALIC
VEIN

Figure 5–1. Veins of the antecubital space are recommended as a site of first choice because they can be cannulated without interrupting CPR. Drugs are given IV push, followed by a 20-mL bolus of normal saline and elevation of the extremity. These actions speed delivery of agents to the central circulation.

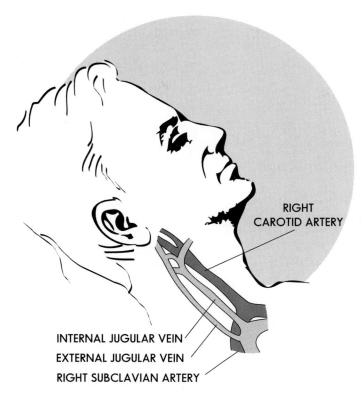

RIGHT
CAROTID ARTERY

INTERNAL JUGULAR VEIN
EXTERNAL JUGULAR VEIN
RIGHT SUBCLAVIAN ARTERY

Figure 5–2. The external jugular veins are also considered a site of first choice during ACLS. They are favored because of their proximity to the central circulation. Unfortunately, cannulation often requires interruption of intubation.

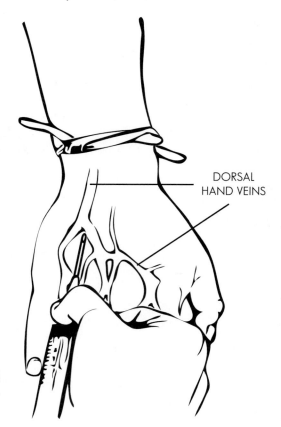

DORSAL
HAND VEINS

Figure 5–3. The veins on the dorsum of the hand are smaller and subject to collapse during cardiac arrest. In the stable patient, however, this is generally an acceptable site.

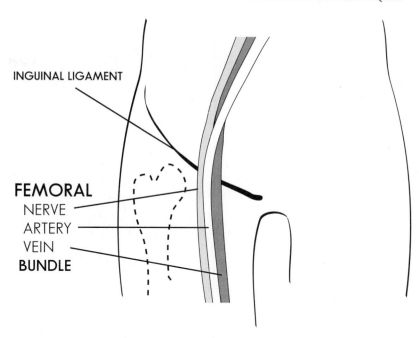

INGUINAL LIGAMENT

FEMORAL
NERVE
ARTERY
VEIN
BUNDLE

Figure 5–4. The femoral vein is large and does not collapse easily. Unfortunately, it is located below the diaphragm and thus receives very little blood flow during CPR. Unless this site is used to access the central circulation, it is *not* recommended for use during ACLS.

The Femoral Vein

Unless the femoral vein (Figure 5–4) is to be cannulated by a catheter long enough to reach the central circulation, this site is *not* recommended for use during ACLS. The reason is that even with adequately performed compressions, little venous blood flow occurs in sites located below the diaphragm. Thus, drugs administered from this site are not felt to adequately reach the central circulation.

The Saphenous Vein

In general, the saphenous vein (Figure 5–5) is the *least* desirable site for obtaining peripheral venous access during CPR. Reasons for this include:

- It is located below the diaphragm. Thus, drugs are not felt to reach the central circulation.
- The risk of *phlebitis* at this site is reportedly high even when isotonic solutions are used.

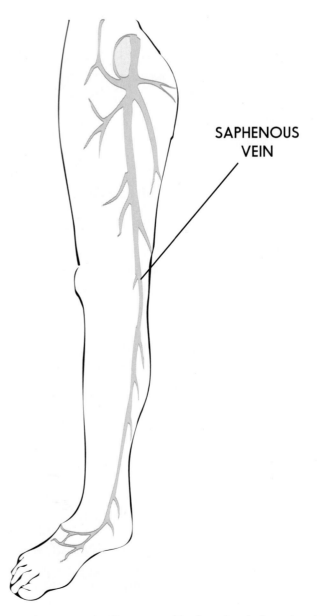

SAPHENOUS
VEIN

Figure 5–5. The saphenous vein. Because of its location below the diaphragm and its associated incidence of phlebitis, this site is not recommended during ACLS.

BIBLIOGRAPHY

1. Aitkenhead AR. Drug administration during CPR: What route? Resuscitation 1991;22:191–195
2. American Heart Association, Emergency Cardiac Care Committee and Subcommittees. Guidelines for cardiopulmonary resuscitation and emergency cardiac care. JAMA 1992;268:2171–2295
3. American Heart Association. Textbook of advanced cardiac life support. Dallas, TX: American Heart Association, 1994

4. American Heart Association. Instructor's manual for advanced cardiac life support. Dallas, TX: American Heart Association, 1994

5. Emerman CL, Pinchak AC, Hancock D, Hagen JF. The effect of bolus injection on circulation times during cardiac arrest. Am J Emerg Med 1009;8:190–193

6. Hess D, Alagar R. Methods of emergency drug administration. Respir Care 1995;40:498–514

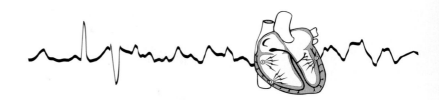

6. Electrocardiology

TYPES OF MYOCARDIAL CELLS

It is important to review the anatomic and physiologic features of myocardial working and electrical system cells as they relate to ACLS.

Myocardial Working Cells

Found in the myocardium, these cells possess the ability to contract. When their cell membranes become depolarized by an electrical impulse or *action potential,* they shorten and then return to their original length. When this happens synchronously, as in a normal heartbeat, the heart functions as a pump and the body's organ systems are perfused.

Electrical System Cells

Working cells are depolarized by an electrical impulse. The twin functions of the heart's electrical system cells are to generate this potential and to rapidly deliver it to the working cells.

The ability to act as a pacemaker and form an action potential is known as *automaticity*. The cells of this system are able to distribute this electrical charge because they possess the quality of *conductivity*.

The structures of the heart's electrical system are illustrated in Figure 6–1. Under normal circumstances, the action potential is generated in the *sinus node* and then distributed throughout the myocardium.

As pictured, the heart's electrical system consists of the following structures.

The Sinus Node

This structure has the fastest rate of automaticity. That is, it generates action potentials more rapidly than other pacemaker cells in the electrical system. With its inherent rate of 60 to 100/min, the sinus node is the dominant pacemaker of the heart.

Internodal Pathways

After its origination in the sinus node, the action potential travels through internodal tracts causing the atrial myocardium to discharge and contract.

The AV Node

After atrial depolarization and contraction, the electrical impulse travels to the AV node. At this grouping of fibers, the impulse is delayed for approxi-

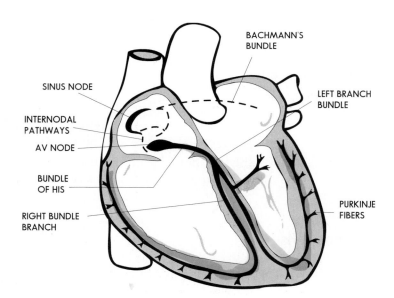

Figure 6–1. The structure of the heart's electrical system.

mately 0.10 second. In the context of ACLS, this pause has the following beneficial effects:

- Ensures ventricular filling at high rates.
- Blockade of ectopic potentials in atrial flutter and atrial fibrillation. This functions to prevent a rapid ventricular response.

Both ischemia and drugs with a negative *dromotropic* effect can cause slowing of conduction through the AV node. When this occurs, first-, second-, or even third-degree AV block may result.

Bundle of His

Also known as the *common bundle*, this structure begins just below the AV node and extends to the superior edge of the interventricular septum. Ischemia can cause blockade to occur at the His bundle level. Because it is not innervated by autonomic fibers, drugs do not affect conduction through this structure.

The Right and Left Bundle Branches

Bifurcating at the top of the interventricular septum, these two major conduction pathways deliver the action potential simultaneously to their respective ventricles. Like the common bundle, bundle branch conduction disturbances cannot be caused or treated by pharmacologic agents.

The Purkinje Fibers

The terminal ends of the bundle branches, these fibers extend throughout the ventricular myocardium. The Purkinje fibers of both right and left ventricles receive their action potential at the same time. Conduction through these fibers is rapid. Thus, under normal circumstances, both ventricles are depolarized and contract simultaneously.

PROPERTIES OF MYOCARDIAL CELLS

Between them, the two types of myocardial cells discussed above possess three properties.

Contractility

Only working cells exhibit this characteristic. Physiologists use the term *inotropicity* to refer to the force of contraction.

Drugs such as epinephrine, dopamine, and dobutamine are said to have a *positive inotropic* effect. In the setting of ACLS, ischemia and acidosis are potent *negative inotropes.*

Conductivity

Both myocardial working cells and electrical system cells possess this ability. As might be imagined however, the electrical system is able to conduct potentials much faster than working cells.

Automaticity

This is the ability to act as a pacemaker by generating action potentials. Only cells within the electrical system have this ability. There are three groups of cells within this system that exhibit important pacemaker activity. They and their inherent rate of automaticity are detailed in Table 6–1.

Sinus Node Pacemakers

As can be noted in Table 6–1, the pacemaker cells located in the sinus node have the fastest rate of automaticity. This structure is the heart's dominant pacemaker. It is also under the control of the autonomic nervous system. Stimulation as occurs under the following circumstances causes the rate of sinus node impulse formation to increase:

- Sympathomimetic drugs
- Parasympatholytic drugs
- Hypoxia

Conversely, decreasing sympathetic activity or ischemic injury to the sinus node can result in sinus bradycardia.

Escape Pacemakers

Junctional pacemakers, located in the AV node, and ventricular pacemakers, located in the Purkinje fibers, have inherent rates of automaticity substantially slower than that of the sinus node. Consequently, they normally do not get a chance to "fire."

However, should the sinus node be slowed, they will act as "escape" or back-up pacemakers. Thus, should the sinus rate fall below 60/min, a

TABLE 6–1. INHERENT RATES OF AUTOMATICITY FOR THE MAJOR MYOCARDIAL PACEMAKERS.

PACEMAKER LOCATION	INHERENT/ESCAPE RATE
Sinus Node	60–100/min.
AV Junctional Tissues	40–50/min.
Ventricular/Purkinje Tissues	Less than 40/min.

junctional escape beat may occur. In a similar fashion, if the rate falls below 40/min, a *ventricular escape beat* will provide backup.

THE ELECTROCARDIOGRAM

Monitoring and Measurements

The electrocardiogram (ECG) is a graphic recording of the heart's electrical activity. Most ECG monitoring systems combine paper strip recordings with a cathode ray screen.

The electrical activity that occurs as the heart contracts and releases is described in terms of six waves. These deflections have been arbitrarily named P, Q, R, S, T, and U.

Additionally, clinicians describe four "segments" or "intervals" within the electrical cycle itself. These are the PR interval, QRS interval, ST segment, and QT segment. These are illustrated in Figure 6–2.

ACLS and other health care providers communicate or "chart" a patient's electrocardiologic status using graphed ECG paper. An example of standard ECG paper appears in Figure 6–3. Please note that the vertical axis is used to measure voltage, whereas the horizontal axis measures time.

Also note in Figure 6–3 the use of the *calibration standard.* This is done periodically to ensure the accuracy of the electrocardiograph machine. The operator activates the proper control whereby the device emits a 1.0-mV electrical impulse to the system which typically lasts for 0.20 seconds. The graphic recording should then register this impulse as a three-sided, rectangular-shaped deflection exactly 10 mm high and 5 mm in length. Figure 6–4 shows another view of the ECG graph paper.

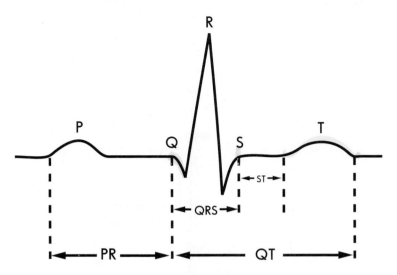

Figure 6–2. The waves and intervals commonly evaluated on the electrocardiogram.

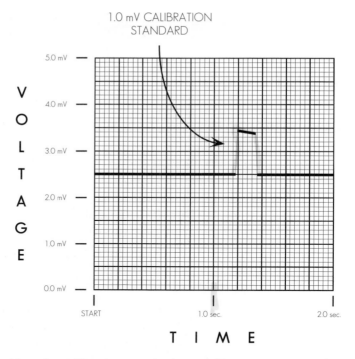

Figure 6–3. Use of a calibration standard to verify measurements of voltage. (Adapted with permission from Meltzer LE, Pinneo R, Kitchell RJ. Intensive Coronary Care, 4th ed. Bowie, MD: Robert J. Brady Co., 1983.)

In Figure 6–4 you will note that the paper is calibrated in *large squares* and *small squares*. These are 5 mm and 1 mm on each side respectively. It should be noted that the electrocardiograph machine which transcribes the rhythm onto paper, operates at a rate of 25 mm/sec.

Using this methodology, a wave or deflection three small squares wide has a duration of 0.12 seconds. Similarly, an interval that is four big squares wide would occur over a 0.80-second span of time.

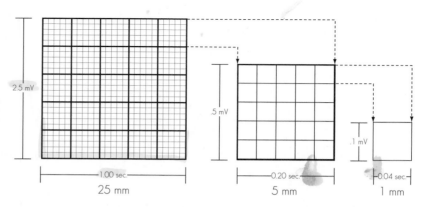

Figure 6–4. The large and small squares used in ECG measurements. (Adapted with permission from Meltzer LE, Pinneo R Kitchell RJ. *Intensive Coronary Care,* 4th ed. Bowie, MD: Robert J. Brady Co., 1983.)

WAVEFORMS OF THE ECG

The P Wave

Depolarization of the atria results in the normally small and somewhat rounded P wave (Figure 6–5). In the chest monitoring leads I, II, and III, the P wave is a positive deflection. P waves should be followed by QRS complexes. Examples of normal and abnormal P waves are seen in Figure 6–6.

The PR Interval

The PR interval as illustrated in Figure 6–7, is measured from the beginning of the P wave to the beginning of the Q wave. In Figure 6–7, it is 0.68 seconds. Measured on actual patients, the normal duration is 0.10 to 0.20 seconds.

The PR interval represents the time it takes the action potential to travel from the sinus node to the ventricles. Thus, a PR interval greater than 0.20 seconds indicates that conduction through AV node has been delayed. This phenomenon can be caused by conduction-slowing drugs such as digitalis, the beta blockers, and the calcium channel blockers.

Examples of normal and abnormal PR intervals are seen in Figure 6–8.

The QRS Complex

The QRS complex (Figure 6–9) represents depolarization of the ventricular muscle mass. It consists of three separate waves.

The Q Wave

In common monitoring leads (I, II, and III), the Q wave is usually a small negative deflection. This wave represents depolarization of the interventricular septum.

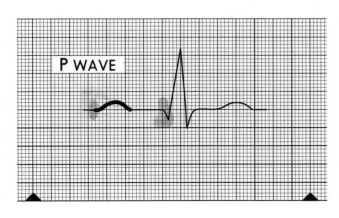

Figure 6–5. The P wave represents depolarization of the atria.

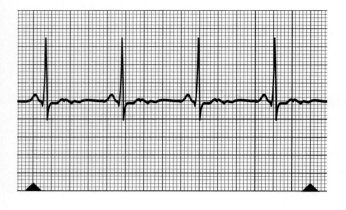

A. NORMAL **P** WAVE

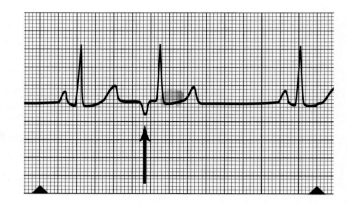

B. INVERTED "JUNCTIONAL" **P** WAVE

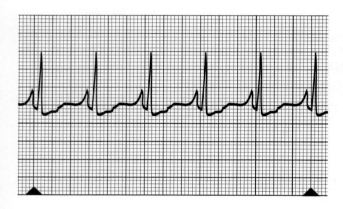

C. PEAKED **P** WAVE TYPICAL OF
   PULMONARY HYPERTENSION

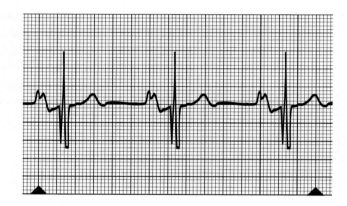

D. BI-PHASIC **P** WAVE SUGGESTIVE OF
   MITRAL VALVULAR DYSFUNCTION

Figure 6–6. Examples of normal and abnormal P waves.

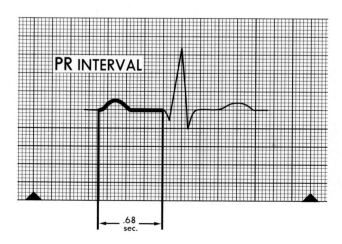

Figure 6–7. The PR interval.

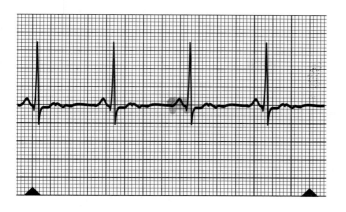

A. NORMAL **PR** INTERVAL

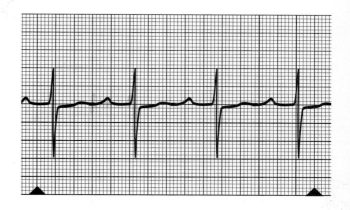

B. WIDENED **PR** INTERVAL OF FIRST DEGREE
AV BLOCK

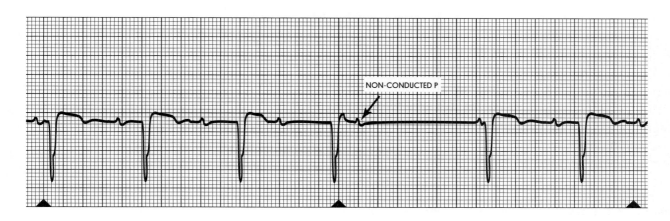

NON-CONDUCTED P

C. GRADUAL WIDENING OF **PR** INTERVAL
SEEN IN SECOND DEGREE TYPE I
AV BLOCK

Figure 6–8. Examples of normal and abnormal PR intervals.

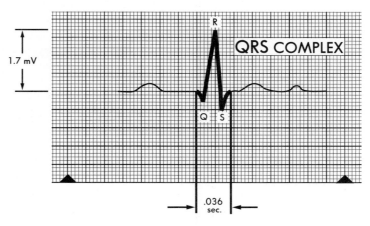

Figure 6–9. The QRS complex.

Following acute myocardial infarction (AMI), Q waves are typically very deep and broad.

The R Wave

This large "spike" represents depolarization of the ventricular muscle mass. It is positive in common monitoring leads (I, II, and III). In lead MCL1 it is a negative deflection.

The S Wave

This normally represents depolarization of the epicardial surface at the base of the ventricles. As illustrated, the QRS is measured from the beginning of the Q wave to the point where the S wave returns to the isoelectric line.

The normal duration of the QRS complex is 0.04 to 0.12 second. In Figure 6–10, please note the fact that normal QRS complexes may vary in shape but are still less than 0.12 seconds. Also note that supraventricular complexes illustrated are typically less than 0.12 seconds. This is because they are conducted through the speedy ventricular conduction system.

An exception, seen in Figure 6–10D is the wide QRS complex of bundle branch block. Here, even though the impulse is supraventricular in origin, the complex is wide due to non-conduction through one of the bundle branches.

Figure 6–11 contains examples of wide QRS complexes. The origin of these impulses is *not* supraventricular. Thus, the resultant complexes are not only broad but often bizarre in appearance. This is because impulses that originate in ventricular pacemaker cells must be conducted slowly through myocardial working cells rather than rapidly through specialized conduction pathways.

The ST Segment

The ST segment represents the period of time between the end of ventricular depolarization and the beginning of ventricular depolarization. As illustrated in Figures 6–12 and 6–13A, the ST segment is normally an isoelectric straight line between the QRS and the T wave. An upward-sloping ST as noted in Figure 6–13B is *not* considered abnormal.

In contrast, *horizontal* and *downward*-sloping ST depression (Figures 6-13C and D) are not normal. These ECG findings often represent myocardial ischemia. Their presence is used to confirm diagnoses of angina pectoris and exercise intolerance.

Myocardial injury, which accompanies and often precedes acute myocardial infarction, will also cause changes in the ST segment. Typical abnormalities indicative of acute myocardial injury are seen in Figure 6–14.

Seen in Figure 6–14A, the "fireman's hat" type is a common example of ST segment elevation. Also common are coved "tombstone"-like elevations noted in Figure 6–14B. A less frequent manifestation of myocardial in-

QRS COMPLEXES OF SUPRAVENTRICULAR ORIGIN

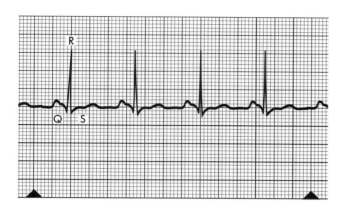

A. NORMAL QRS

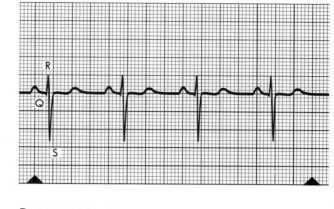

B. NORMAL QRS

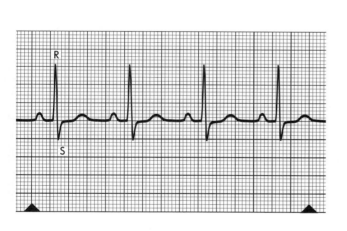

C. NORMAL QRS

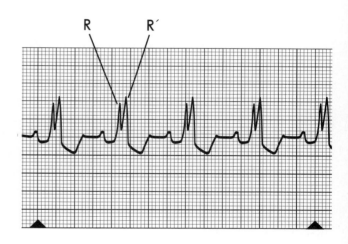

D. "M" SHAPED COMPLEX OF BUNDLE BRANCH BLOCK

Figure 6–10. When the impulse is generated above the ventricles, the QRS complex is typically narrow. An exception is bundle branch block.

jury (Figure 6–14C) are *reciprocal* ST segment depressions. These are a mirror image of elevated ST segments.

The T Wave

The T wave depicted in Figure 6–15 represents ventricular *repolarization* or recovery. Slightly larger and more rounded in appearance than the P wave, it follows the ST segment just described. A normal T wave is depicted in Figure 6–16A.

WIDE QRS COMPLEXES OF VENTRICULAR ORIGIN

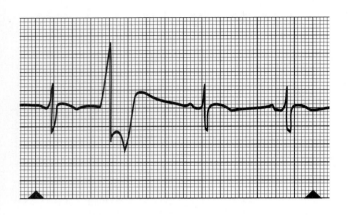

A. UNIFOCAL **PVC**

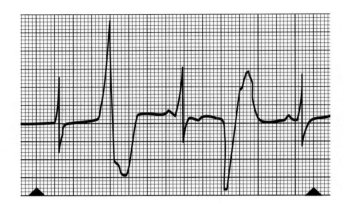

B. MULTIFOCAL **PVC**

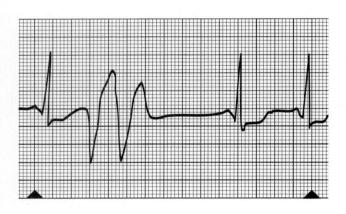

C. PAIRED **PVC**'S

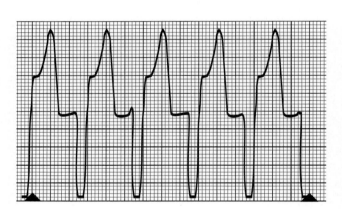

D. VENTRICULAR TACHYCARDIA

Figure 6–11. Wide and bizarre complexes result when impulses of ventricular origin are conducted through myocardial instead of conduction system cells.

Peaked T waves (Figure 6–16B) are an indicator of hyperkalemia but may be seen in patients with normal potassium levels.

Inverted T waves that are sharply pointed and look like an *arrowhead* are a classic sign of the ischemia that accompanies an acute myocardial infarction. An example can be seen in Figure 6–16C.

The QT Interval

The QT interval (Figure 6–17) represents the duration of both depolarization and repolarization. The QT interval has a normal range of 0.24 to 0.40

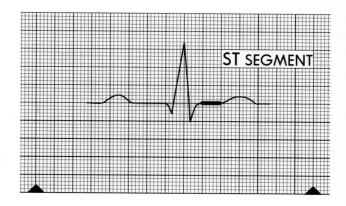

Figure 6–12. Representation of a normal isoelectric ST segment.

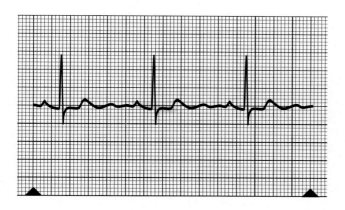

A. NORMAL ISOLECTRIC **ST** SEGMENT

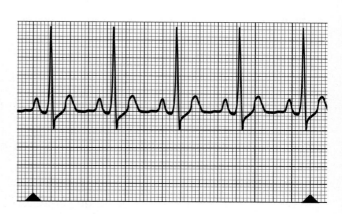

B. NORMAL UPWARD SLOPING **ST** SEGMENT

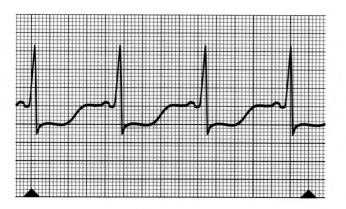

C. HORIZONTAL **ST** DEPRESSION OF ISCHEMIA & ANGINA PECTORIS

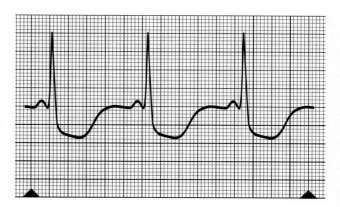

D. DOWNWARD SLOPING **ST** DEPRESSION OF ISCHEMIA & ANGINA PECTORIS

Figure 6–13. Depressed and normal ST segments. (Adapted with permission from Meltzer LE, Pinneo R, Kitchell RJ. Intensive Coronary Care, 4th ed. Bowie, MD: Robert J. Brady Co., 1983.)

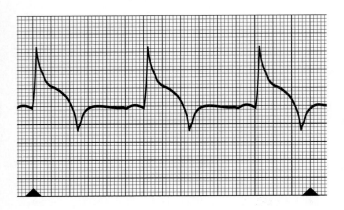

A. "FIREMAN'S HAT" **ST** ELEVATION
TYPICAL OF ACUTE MYOCARDIAL
INJURY

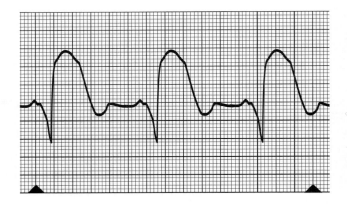

B. COVED ELEVATION OF **ST** SEGMENT
SEEN WITH ACUTE MYOCARDIAL INJURY

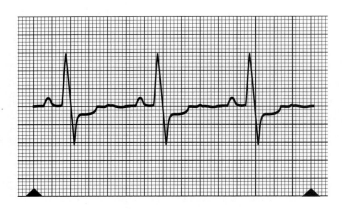

C. RECIPROCAL "FIREMAN'S HAT"
ST SEGMENT DEPRESSION OF
ACUTE MYOCARDIAL INJURY

Figure 6–14. ST segment changes associated with acute myocardial injury. (Adapted with permission from Meltzer LE, Pinneo R, Kitchell RJ. Intensive Coronary Care, 4th ed. Bowie, MD: Robert J. Brady Co., 1983.)

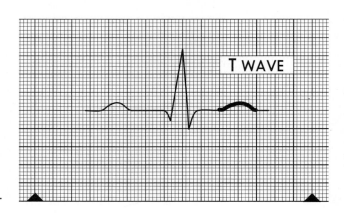

Figure 6–15. The T wave.

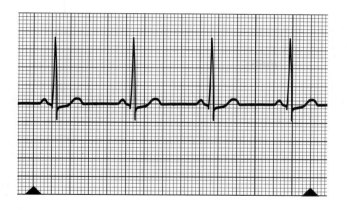

A. NORMAL T WAVE

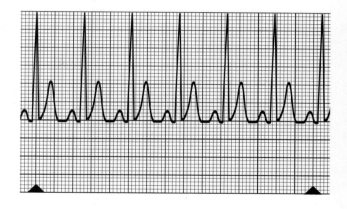

B. PEAKED T WAVE MAY ACCOMPANY
ELECTROLYTE DISTURBANCES

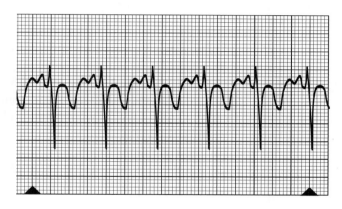

C. INVERTED T WAVES OF ACUTE
MYOCARDIAL ISCHEMIA

Figure 6–16. Examples of T waves.

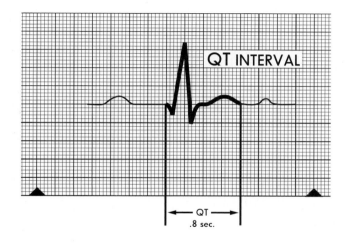

Figure 6–17. A drawing of the QT interval.

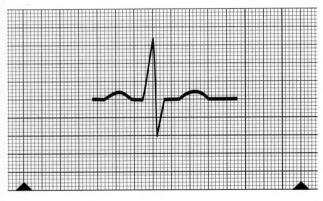

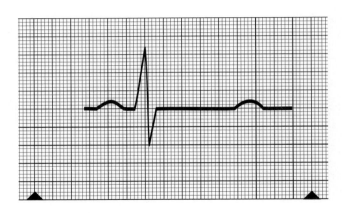

A. SHORTENED **QT** INTERVAL THAT OFTEN ACCOMPANIES HYPERCALCEMIA

B. PROLONGED **QT** INTERVAL ASSOCIATED WITH HYPOCALCEMIA AND PROCAINAMIDE OVERUSAGE

Figure 6–18. Representations of narrow and widened QT intervals.

seconds. Shortened QT intervals are known to accompany hypercalcemia. A drawing of this appears in Figure 6–18A.

A more common occurrence to the ACLS provider (Figure 6–18B) is the widening of the QT interval that can accompany procainamide administration. Widening of the QT intervals is also felt to forewarn the polymorphic form of ventricular tachycardia known as Torsade de pointes.

The U Wave

Often not visible on the ECG, this small positive deflection can be due to repolarization of the Purkinje system. Of uncertain significance, U waves (Figures 6–19 and 6–20) are associated with a variety of factors. Among them are hypokalemia, digitalis administration, and ventricular premature beats.

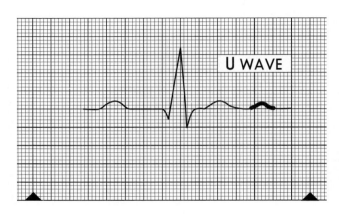

Figure 6–19. Drawing of the U wave.

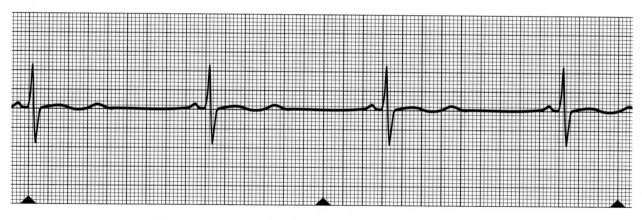

Figure 6–20. Sinus bradycardia with prominent U waves.

ELECTROPHYSIOLOGY

The electrical cycle of the heart consists of myocardial working cells becoming *depolarized* and then undergoing *repolarization*. Electrocardiologically, this corresponds to the appearance of the QRS complex and the subsequent T wave. Physiologically, depolarization occurs when positively charged *sodium* ions rapidly enter the working myocardial cell. Repolarization is essentially the reverse process as positively charged ions, *potassium* in this case, leave the cell.

As Figure 6–21 illustrates, this process occurs in five phases. Also note that the second half of phase 3 is termed the *relative refractory period* of the electrophysiologic cycle.

The sequence of events of the five phases shown in Figure 6–21 are as follows.

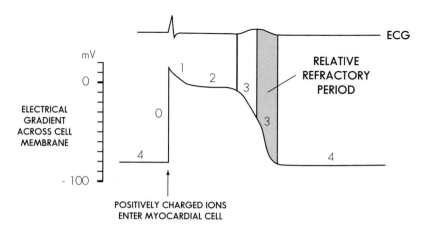

Figure 6–21. The electrophysiology of the depolarization/repolarization cycle. Note the relationship between the ECG and the various phases of this cycle.

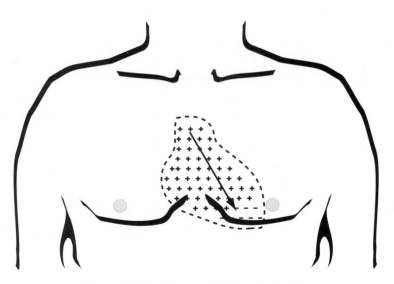

Figure 6–22. Myocardial depolarization.

Phase 0: Depolarization

At the onset of phase 0, fast channels in myocardial cell membrane open causing *sodium* ions to rapidly enter the cell resulting in the QRS complex. As seen in Figure 6–21, this causes the electrical charge inside the cells to rise from its resting (polarized) value of -80 to -90 mV to a positive charge of 10 to 20 mV.

Figure 6–22 is a graphic representation of depolarization. The action potential is a wave of electrical excitation that sweeps through the myocardium from top to apex along the axis indicated by the arrow. Of course in actuality the atria and ventricles are discharged at separate times.

Figure 6–23 shows electrode placement positions used for defib-

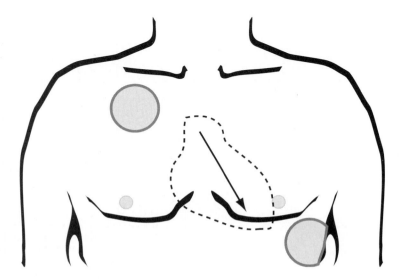

Figure 6–23. Electrode placement positions for defibrillation.

rillation. Note that the electrodes are to be placed along the axis of depolarization (Figures 6–22 and 6–23).

Phases 1 and 2: Slow Repolarization

Here the cells remain depolarized or positively charged as seen in Figures 6–23 and 6–24. At the same time, the charge inside the cell begins to become less positive.

Phases 1 and 2 correspond to the ST segment of the ECG.

Phase 3: Rapid Repolarization

During phase 3, positively charged *potassium* ions leave the cells causing the charge inside them to become negative once again. As Figure 6–21 illustrates, phase 3 corresponds to the T wave on the ECG.

It also depicts the latter portion of phase 3, which translates into the downslope of the T wave. This part of phase 3 is termed the *relative refractory period* of the electric cycle.

During the *absolute refractory period*, pictured in Figure 6–25, the myocardial cells are positively charged. Thus, if an action potential were to occur, the cells, already depolarized, would not respond to the impulse.

However, this is not the case during the latter portion of phase 3. Here the cells, as the wave of repolarization sweeps upward, are a mixture of positive and negative charges (Figure 6–26).

This is the so-called *vulnerable period* of the cardiac cycle. Because of the mixture of cell charges the myocardium is *relatively refractory*.

Thus, an action potential such as occurs when a PVC falls on the

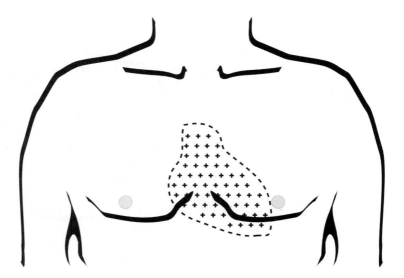

Figure 6–24. During phases 1 and 2, the electrical charge inside the cells remains positive.

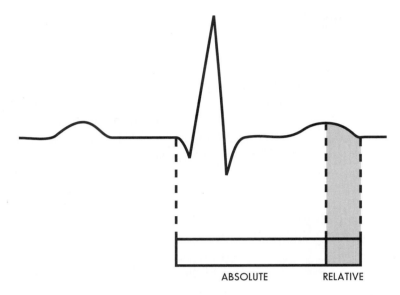

Figure 6–25. The absolute and relative refractory periods of the cardiac cycle.

downslope of the T wave can depolarize cells that are negatively charged. Cells that are positively charged would still be refractory!

In this case, ventricular fibrillation can be precipitated. An example of this, the "R on T phenomenon," is illustrated in Figure 6–27.

Phase 4: Polarization

Here the cells return to their resting charge of –80 to –90 mV (Figures 6–21 and 6–28). In this state, they are said to be *polarized*.

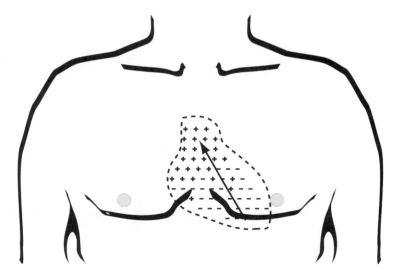

Figure 6–26. The relative refractory period with its mixture of negatively and positively charged cells.

T   QRS   PVC ᴏɴ T

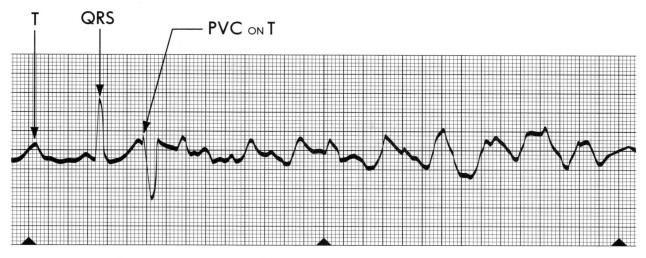

Figure 6–27. The R on T phenomenon precipitating ventricular fibrillation.

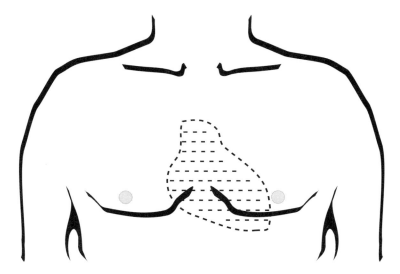

Figure 6–28. Phase 4 of the electric cycle. Here the cells are polarized or negatively charged.

ECG MONITORING DURING ACLS

The Chest Leads

There are three standard chest leads: lead I (Figures 6–29 and 6–30), lead II (Figures 6–31 and 6–32), and lead III (Figures 6–33 and 6–34). These and their electrode placement positions are illustrated on the next few pages. Also pictured is the modified chest lead I (MCL1) (Figures 6–35 and 6–36). This latter lead is used during ACLS because it better allows for administration of electrical therapy such as transcutaneous pacing, and defibrillation.

In selecting a monitoring lead, the most important considerations are practical ones.

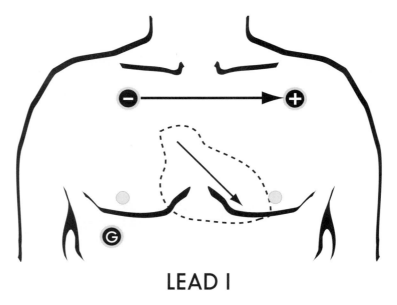

LEAD I

Figure 6–29. Electrode placement for lead I.

- Is R wave amplitude great enough to trigger the rate alarms?
- Is the precordium accessible should electrical therapy be required?
- Can electrodes be placed and maintained without artifact?
- Is the monitor being used for the proper purpose? It is more practical to monitor the QRS complex than to use the chest leads to interpret the extent of myocardial injury and ischemia.

Lead I

The electrode placement positions (Figure 6–29) for chest lead I are stated below.

- Positive electrode below left clavicle.
- Negative electrode below right clavicle.
- Ground below right pectoral muscle.

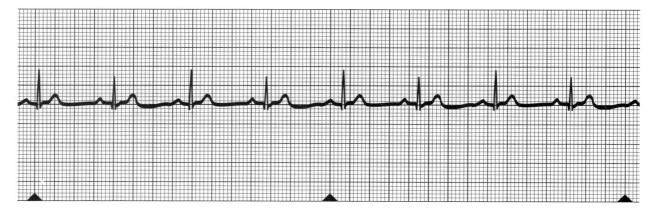

Figure 6–30. Normal sinus rhythm recorded in lead I.

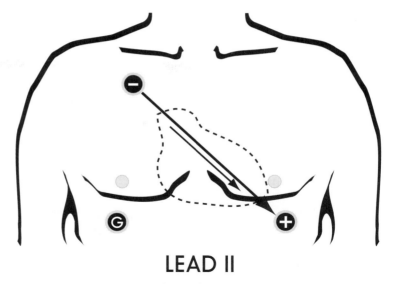

LEAD II

Figure 6–31. Electrode position for lead II.

Figure 6–30 shows an ECG recorded in lead I. In this lead, P waves and R wave are positive, but are often not as prominent as in the other chest leads.

Lead II

The electrode placement positions (Figure 6–31) for chest lead II are stated below.

- Positive electrode below left pectoral muscle.
- Negative electrode below the right clavicle.
- Ground below right pectoral muscle.

R waves are usually most prominent in lead II (Figure 6–32). This is because the direction of polarity from negative to positive is parallel to that of normal depolarization of the ventricular muscle mass.

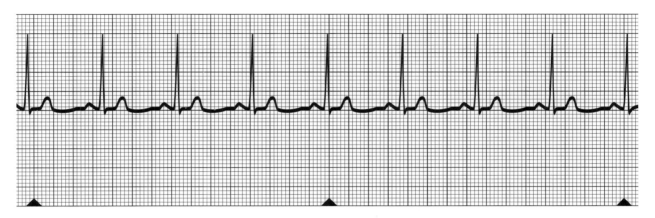

Figure 6–32. Normal sinus rhythm recorded in lead II.

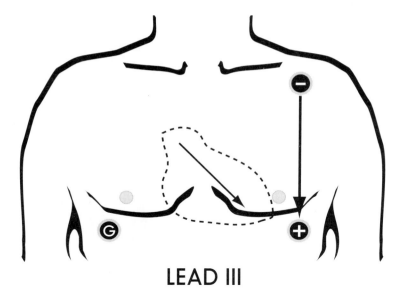

LEAD III

Figure 6–33. Electrode placement for lead III.

Lead III

The electrode placement positions (Figure 6–33) for chest lead III are stated below.

- Positive electrode below left pectoral muscle.
- Negative electrode below left clavicle.
- Ground below right pectoral muscle.

Figure 6–34 shows an ECG recorded in lead III. Note that both P waves and R waves are positive when recorded in this lead.

Modified Chest Lead I

The electrode placement positions (Figure 6–35) for chest lead MCL1 are stated below.

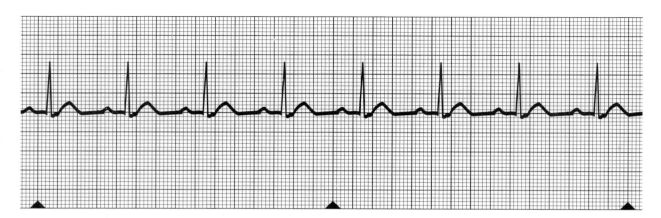

Figure 6–34. Normal sinus rhythm recorded in lead III.

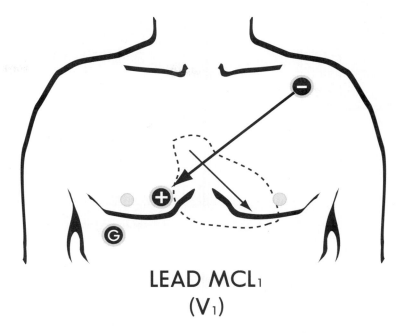

LEAD MCL₁
(V₁)

Figure 6–35. Electrode placement for lead MCL1.

- Positive electrode to the right of the sternum at the fourth intercostal space.
- Negative electrode below left clavicle.
- Ground below left pectoral muscle.

Lead MCL1 (Figure 6–35) is frequently chosen during ACLS because it does not interfere with electrical therapy. P waves tend to be prominent in this lead because the positive electrode is closer to the atria. R waves are inverted because the direction of polarity is 90° from normal depolarization. Figure 6–36 shows an ECG recorded in lead MCL1. Please note the negative deflection of the R wave.

The 12-Lead ECG

Discussion of the 12-lead ECG is beyond the scope of a basic ACLS course. For the sake of completeness, only the briefest review will appear here.

As Figure 6–37 illustrates, the 12-lead ECG is easily performed. All that is required is to attach ten electrodes (six over the precordium, and four to the extremities) and then push the monitoring device's "start" control. The electrocardiograph then selects the proper combination of positive, negative, and ground electrodes for each lead and subsequently provides the operator with a 12-lead electrocardiogram.

This recording consists of the following views of the heart's electrical activity.

Six precordial leads. These view the heart in a horizontal plane from each of the six electrode placement sites on the patient's precordium (Figure 6–37).

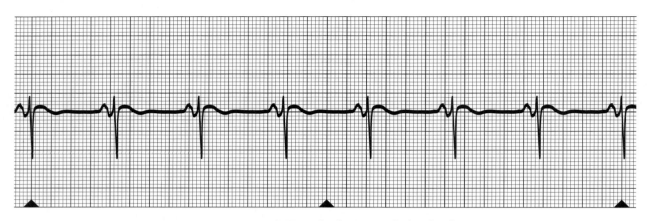

Figure 6–36. Normal sinus rhythm recorded in lead MCL1.

V_1 and V_2: View the right ventricle.
V_3 and V_4: View the interventricular septum.
V_5 and V_6: View the left ventricle.

Three standard leads. These view the heart's electrical activity in a frontal plane. Each lead is bipolar, that is, has a positive and negative electrode. The electrocardiograph in these leads is a recording of the potential difference between these electrodes.

Lead I: Right arm is negative and left arm is positive.
Lead II: Right arm is negative and left foot is positive.
Lead III: Left arm is negative and left foot is positive.

Three augmented leads. These use the same three limbs as the standard leads except in different electrical combinations. These leads are called augmented leads because the electrical potential measured is very small and must be amplified or augmented by the electrocardiograph.

Lead AVR: Right arm is positive.
Lead AVL: Left arm is positive.
Lead AVF: Left foot is positive.

Figure 6–38 illustrates a 12-lead ECG showing extensive acute anterior wall infarction. As will be discussed in Chapter 8, electrocardiographic signs of AMI include deep, wide Q waves, elevated ST segments, and sharply inverted T waves.

MEASUREMENT OF CARDIAC RATE

There are many ways to determine cardiac rate, but in the interest of simplicity, we will only deal with two of the most clinically useful methods.

THE TWELVE-LEAD ECG

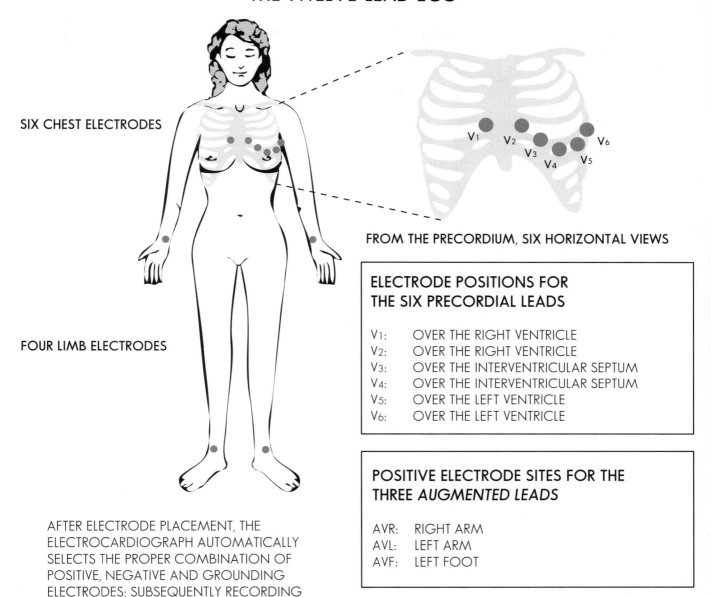

SIX CHEST ELECTRODES

FOUR LIMB ELECTRODES

FROM THE PRECORDIUM, SIX HORIZONTAL VIEWS

ELECTRODE POSITIONS FOR THE SIX PRECORDIAL LEADS

V_1:	OVER THE RIGHT VENTRICLE
V_2:	OVER THE RIGHT VENTRICLE
V_3:	OVER THE INTERVENTRICULAR SEPTUM
V_4:	OVER THE INTERVENTRICULAR SEPTUM
V_5:	OVER THE LEFT VENTRICLE
V_6:	OVER THE LEFT VENTRICLE

POSITIVE ELECTRODE SITES FOR THE THREE *AUGMENTED LEADS*

AVR:	RIGHT ARM
AVL:	LEFT ARM
AVF:	LEFT FOOT

AFTER ELECTRODE PLACEMENT, THE ELECTROCARDIOGRAPH AUTOMATICALLY SELECTS THE PROPER COMBINATION OF POSITIVE, NEGATIVE AND GROUNDING ELECTRODES; SUBSEQUENTLY RECORDING THE TWELVE-LEAD ELECTROCARDIOGRAPH.

ELECTRODE COMBINATION FOR THE THREE *STANDARD LEADS*

I :	RIGHT ARM NEGATIVE - LEFT ARM POSITIVE
II :	RIGHT ARM NEGATIVE - LEFT FOOT POSITIVE
III:	LEFT ARM NEGATIVE - LEFT FOOT POSITIVE

Figure 6–37. Essential features of the 12-lead ECG.

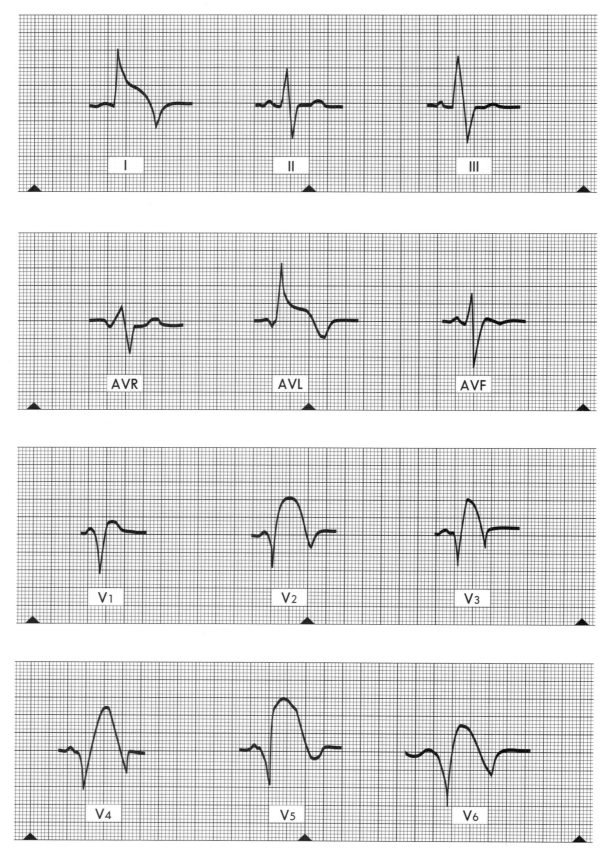

Figure 6–38. 12-lead ECG showing extensive acute anterior wall infarction. (Adapted with permission from Meltzer LE, Pinneo R, Kitchell RJ. Intensive Coronary Care, 4th ed. Bowie, MD: Robert J. Brady Co., 1983.)

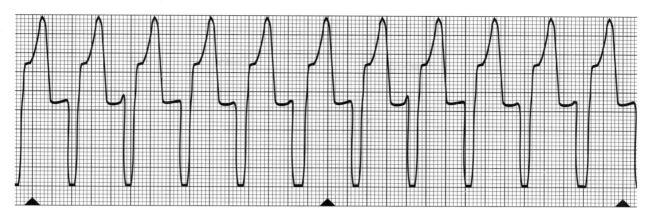

Figure 6–39. ECG recording with a rate slightly over 100/min.

The Six-second Method

ECG paper has "time markings" every three seconds. To arrive at an accurate bedside approximation of rate, the provider should count the number of R–R intervals between two of these three-second marks (six seconds) and then multiply this number by 10. This will yield a fairly accurate rate measurement.

In Figure 6–39, there are just slightly more than ten R–R intervals in the span of six seconds illustrated. Thus, the rate is between 100 and 105/min.

The Two-beat Method

This is the quickest and easiest method for most providers. Unfortunately, it is not accurate when the R–R interval is irregular. The technique is as follows:

- Count the number of large (5 mm) squares between two R waves.
- Divide 300 by that number.
- The answer will be an acceptably accurate rate determination.

Stated mathematically, the formula is:

$$\frac{300}{\#\ \text{Large Squares}} = \text{Cardiac Rate}$$

Applying this method to Figure 6–37, one is able to count slightly less than three large squares between R waves. Plugging this number into the equation, we get:

$$\frac{300}{2.9\ \text{Large Squares}} = 103/\text{min}$$

Figure 6–40 illustrates the basis for this method.

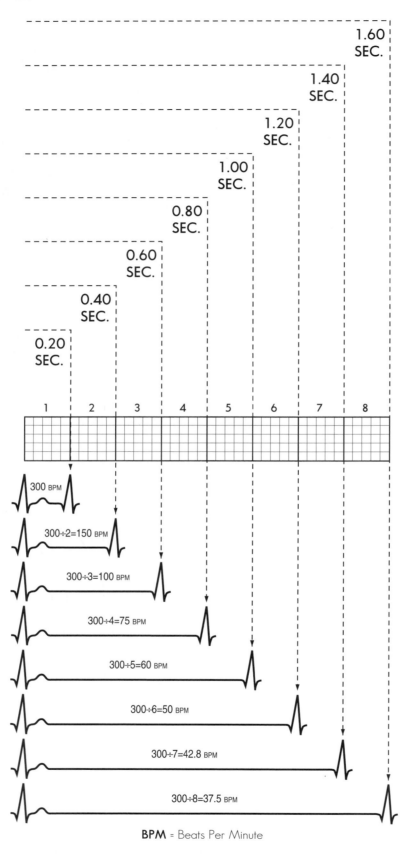

BPM = Beats Per Minute

Figure 6–40. Diagrammatic representation of the two-beat method of rate measurement.

BIBLIOGRAPHY

1. American Heart Association, Emergency Cardiac Care Committee and Subcommittees. Guidelines for cardiopulmonary resuscitation and emergency cardiac care. JAMA 1992;268:2171–2295
2. American Heart Association. Textbook of advanced cardiac life support. Dallas, TX: American Heart Association, 1994
3. American Heart Association. Instructor's manual for advanced cardiac life support. Dallas, TX: American Heart Association, 1994
4. Meltzer LE, Pinneo R, and Kitchell JR. Intensive Coronary Care, 4th ed. Norwalk, CT: Appleton & Lange, 1983.

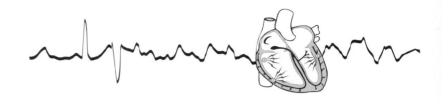

7. Electrocardiographic Signs of Ischemia Injury and Infarct

ATHEROSCLEROTIC HEART DISEASE

Of the two million or so deaths every year in the United States, approximately 25% are the result of acute myocardial infarction (AMI). Strokes are a distant second cause of death, claiming 150,000 victims each year.

Pathologists have determined that almost all episodes of myocardial infarction are the result of progressive atherosclerotic heart disease (ASHD). It is commonly accepted that by the age of 50, the overwhelming majority of men in the United States have some degree of ASHD.

It is rare for ASHD to produce symptoms. Indeed, fully 20% of victims who die as a result of AMI are asymptomatic prior to the event.

The pathophysiology of ASHD involves the formation of cholesterol-laden atheromas just beneath the coronary arterial endothelium. With time, atheromas both grow and undergo calcification. This results in coronary arteries that are both narrowed and sclerotic. An acute ischemic event is precipitated when one of these calcified plaques ruptures into the lumen of an artery.

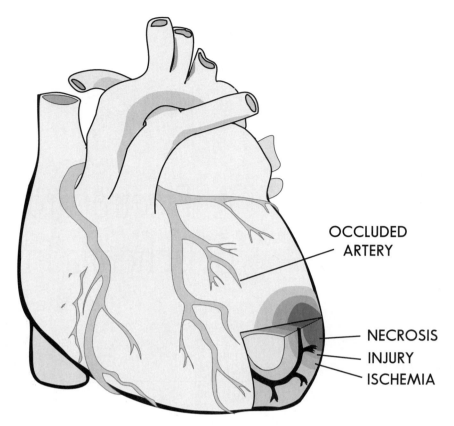

OCCLUDED ARTERY

NECROSIS

INJURY

ISCHEMIA

Figure 7–1. The three zones of cellular pathology associated with acute myocardial infarction. (Adapted with permission from Meltzer LE, Pinneo R, Kitchell RJ. Intensive Coronary Care, 4th ed. Bowie, MD: Robert J. Brady Co., 1983.)

The jagged surfaces of plaque cause circulating platelets to form a clot at the site of the rupture. This thrombus further occludes the affected artery and may completely block it. The result is that blood flow slows or even stops.

Subsequently, the myocardial cells supplied by the occluded coronary artery undergo one or more of the following pathologic changes. As Figure 7–1 illustrates, the lesion of AMI actually consists of three somewhat distinct zones.

- **Necrosis.** This is the central area of dead myocardial cells. The goal of therapeutic interventions is to keep this zone from enlarging.
- **Injury.** Surrounding the necrotic tissues are injured cells. Frequently, pacemaker cells are injured, resulting in *altered automaticity*.
- **Ischemia.** Finally, an *outermost* area of cells are ischemic. That is, they are not perfused or oxygenated adequately.

The presence and, to some extent, the magnitude of each of these areas can be evaluated by analysis of specific changes in the ECG. Accordingly, the ACLS provider can assess the need for, and the success of, measures such as *thrombolytic agents.*

ECG DETERMINATION OF MYOCARDIAL ISCHEMIA

Following occlusion, the cells supplied by that coronary artery *first* become ischemic. As Figure 7–2 illustrates, the classic ECG sign of myocardial ischemia is *inverted and sharply pointed T waves that resemble an arrowhead.*

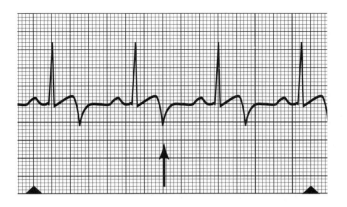

A. NORMAL SINUS RHYTHM WITH INVERTED
   T WAVE

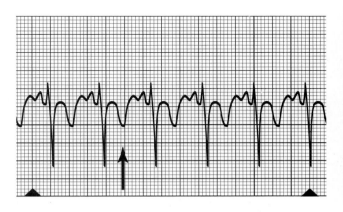

B. SINUS TACHYCARDIA WITH INVERTED
   T WAVE

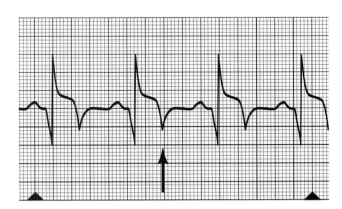

C. INVERTED **T** WAVE WITH **ST** SEGMENT
   ELEVATION AND PRONOUNCED **Q** WAVE

Figure 7–2. Examples of inverted T waves. Inverted T waves that resemble an arrowhead are frequently caused by myocardial ischemia. (Adapted with permission from Meltzer LE, Pinneo R, Kitchell RJ. Intensive Coronary Care, 4th ed. Bowie, MD: Robert J. Brady Co., 1983.)

ECG DETERMINATION OF MYOCARDIAL INJURY

Following ischemia, myocardial injury develops. Altered membrane permeability effects slow repolarization in the electrophysiologic cycle. The result, as Figure 7–3 illustrates, is ST segment elevation.

A definitive diagnosis of myocardial infarction usually cannot be established until some hours have elapsed. Thus, the presence of ST segment elevation greater than 0.1 mV (1 mm) in at least two contiguous leads on a 12-lead ECG is considered evidence that the victim is *myocardially infarcting*.

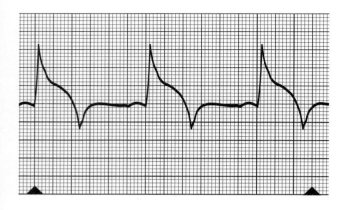

A. "FIREMAN'S HAT" **ST** ELEVATION

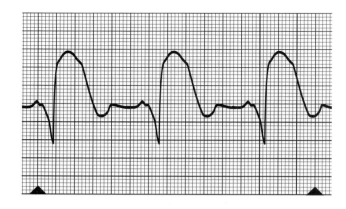

B. COVED ELEVATION OF **ST** SEGMENT

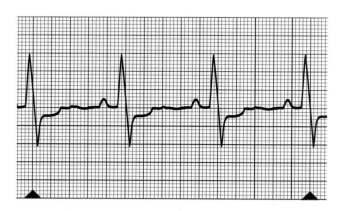

C. RECIPROCAL "FIREMAN'S HAT"
ST SEGMENT DEPRESSION

Figure 7–3. Examples of ST segment elevation. Clinically, ST segment elevation greater than 1 mm (0.1 mV) in at least two contiguous leads on a 12-lead ECG is (subject to physician review) considered evidence that the patient is infarcting and is thus an indication for thrombolytic therapy. (Adapted with permission from Meltzer LE, Pinneo R, Kitchell RJ. Intensive Coronary Care, 4th ed. Bowie, MD: Robert J. Brady Co., 1983.)

The JAMA guidelines state that concluding a patient is myocardially infarcting is a *presumption,* not an actual diagnosis.

In clinical practice, these vital distinctions are left to specially trained physicians. Additionally, the current ACLS instructor's manual states that the discussion of injury versus infarction is beyond the scope of an essential ACLS provider course.

Another reason this determination is subject to physician review is that patients identified as infarcting are candidates for thrombolytic therapy. Thrombolytic agents have revolutionized the treatment of patients with AMI. This class of drugs has the ability to actually reopen blocked coronary arteries. We will present a case history in Chapter 9 demonstrating ECG changes following therapy.

ECG DETERMINATION OF MYOCARDIAL INFARCT

The classic sign of myocardial infarction is the presence of *deep, wide Q waves.* As Figure 7–4 indicates, this is true for acute, recent, and healed myocardial infarction.

Note that the ST segment and T-wave abnormalities disappear over time. This is because injured and ischemic cells that don't undergo necrosis usually heal.

This is not the case with the Q waves of infarction. Because necrotic tissue generates no electrical activity, the deep Q waves that result do not disappear.

Definitive diagnosis of AMI is made on the basis of presence of pathologic Q waves on a 12-lead ECC and serum creatinine phosphokinase isoenzyme studies.

Unfortunately, pronounced Q waves may take hours to develop following AMI. Serum isoenzyme results may also take hours. Neither the patient nor the ACLS provider can afford to wait for these results. This underscores the importance of ST segment monitoring discussed previously.

Thus, patients with ST segment elevation greater than 1 mm in two contiguous leads on a 12-lead ECG are *presumed* to be myocardially infarcting. This person qualifies for thrombolytic therapy despite the absence of pathologic Q waves.

DETERMINING THE LOCATION OF AMI

Similar to evaluating the need for thrombolytic therapy, the subject of determining the location of a myocardial infarction is beyond the scope of an essential ACLS provider course. Consequently, this text will confine itself to presenting the ECG criteria listed in the guidelines.

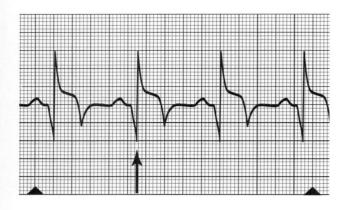

A. ACUTE M.I. NOTE THE SIGNS OF INJURY AND ISCHEMIA

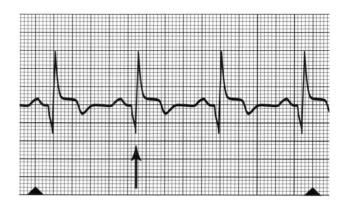

B. RECENT M.I.

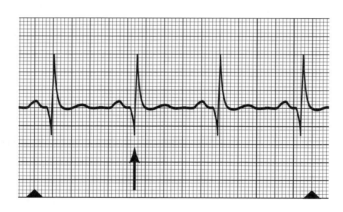

C. HEALED M.I. NOTE RELATIVELY NORMAL ST SEGMENT AND T WAVE

Figure 7–4. The deep, wide Q waves of myocardial infarction. Note that over time, noninfarcted cells undergo healing, as evidenced by the disappearance of abnormal ST segment and T-wave changes.

Criteria for Anterior Wall Infarct/Injury

Occlusion of the anterior descending branch of the left coronary artery is indicated by the following signs on a 12-lead ECG:

- **Injury.** ST segment elevation in leads V_1 through V_4.
- **Infarction.** Pronounced Q waves in leads V_1 through V_4.

Figure 7–5 is a representation of a 12-lead ECG typical of an anterior wall infarction. The presence of inverted T waves signifies that the ischemic event is acute.

The signs of injury exist in V_1 through V_4. They can also be seen in V_5, V_6, I, and AVL. This strongly suggests that the lesion is a large or extensive one.

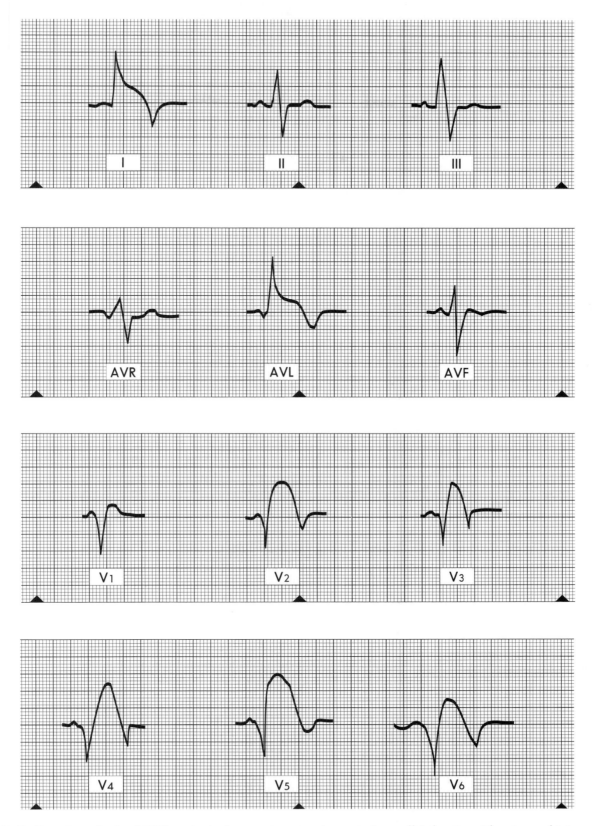

Figure 7–5. Drawing of a lead ECG typical of an acute extensive anterior wall infarction. The signs of injury and infarction are present in leads V_1 through V_4 and additionally in V_5, V_6, I, and AVL. Inverted T waves signify that the lesion is fresh. (Adapted with permission from Meltzer LE, Pinneo R, Kitchell RJ. Intensive Coronary Care, 4th ed. Bowie, MD: Robert J. Brady Co., 1983.)

Criteria for Inferior Wall Infarct/Injury

Occlusion of the right coronary artery is indicated by the following ECG signs:

- **Injury.** ST segment elevation in leads II, III, and AVF.
- **Infarction.** Pronounced Q waves in leads II, III, and AVF.

Criteria for Right Ventricular Infarct/Injury

About 25% of patients with inferior infarcts have right ventricular involvement. Injury and infarction of the right ventricle is identified by pronounced Q waves and ST segment elevations in leads II, III, AVF, plus V_4R.

Criteria for Lateral Wall Infarct/Injury

Characteristic Q waves and ST segment elevation in leads I, AVL, V_5, and V_6.

Criteria for Posterior Infarct/Injury

Characteristic Q waves and reciprocal ST segment depression in leads V_1 and V_2.

BIBLIOGRAPHY

1. American Heart Association, Emergency Cardiac Care Committee and Subcommittees. Guidelines for cardiopulmonary resuscitation and emergency cardiac care. JAMA 1992;268:2171–2295
2. American Heart Association. Textbook of advanced cardiac life support. Dallas, TX: American Heart Association, 1994
3. American Heart Association. Instructor's manual for advanced cardiac life support. Dallas, TX: American Heart Association, 1994
4. Eisenberg MS, Aghababian RV, Bossaert L, Jaffe AS, Ornato JP, Weaver WD. Thrombolytic therapy. Ann Emerg Med 1993;22(Part 2):417–427
5. Junnar RM, Bourdillon PO, Dixon DW, et al. ACC/AHA guidelines for the early management of patients with acute myocardial infarction. Circulation 1990;82: 664–707
6. Meltzer LE, Pinneo R, and Kitchell JR. Intensive Coronary Care, 4th ed. Norwalk CT: Appleton & Lange, 1983

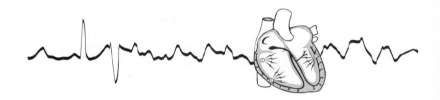

8. Mechanisms of Arrhythmia Formation

THE NORMAL SINUS RHYTHM

The normal electrocardiogram is termed a *normal sinus rhythm.* It is described as a monotonously regular succession of PQRS and T waves occurring at a rate of 60 to 100 per minute. An example of a normal sinus rhythm is seen in Figure 8–1.

Other criteria of a normal sinus rhythm include:

- **Impulse origination in the sinus node.** This is indicated by the presence of normal P waves, each of which is followed by a QRS complex. P waves that are not followed by a QRS complex are termed dropped impulses.

129

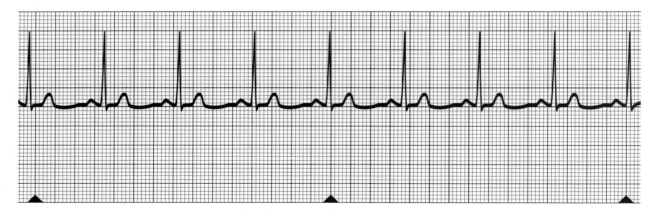

Figure 8–1. Normal sinus rhythm. Note the *monotonously regular* succession of PQRS and T waves.

- **Evidence of normal conduction.** When the PR interval and the QRS complexes are within their normal limits of 0.10 to 0.20 second and 0.04 to 0.12 second, respectively, conduction is said to be normal.

MECHANISMS OF ARRHYTHMIA FORMATION

When a patient's electrocardiogram does not meet the criteria for a normal sinus rhythm, an arrhythmia is said to exist. The term *arrhythmia* means an "absence of rhythm." The similar term *dysrhythmia* means an "abnormality in rhythm." Both terms may be used interchangeably. The editors of most medical journals, including those of the *Journal of the American Medical Association*, use the term arrhythmia almost exclusively. For this reason, this term will be used in this text.

There are three important mechanisms responsible for arrhythmia formation. They can be used to explain the pathophysiology of the lethal and nonlethal arrhythmias for which the ACLS provider is responsible. They are as follows:

- Abnormal sinus node automaticity
- Conduction disturbances
- Ectopic impulse formation

In cardiology, the term *ectopy* is used to describe myocardial contractions that are caused by pacemakers located outside the sinus node. Arrhythmias caused by ectopic pacemakers are of primary concern to the ACLS provider. This is because they are the cause of ventricular fibrillation and ventricular tachycardia.

ABNORMAL SINUS NODE AUTOMATICITY

The sinus node is the dominant pacemaker because it has the fastest rate of automaticity. This group of cells is under the control of the autonomic nervous system. Sympathetic stimulation will accelerate their rate of automaticity. In contrast, parasympathetic dominance will slow impulse formation.

Under normal circumstances, these twin branches of the autonomic nervous system exist in a state of *balanced antagonism.* The result is generation of 60 to 100 action potentials each minute. When sinus node automaticity falls outside these limits, a sinus tachycardia or a sinus bradycardia is said to exist. These arrhythmias are discussed below.

Sinus Tachycardia

When more than 100 impulses per minute are created by the sinus node, the electrocardiographic result is called *sinus tachycardia* (Figure 8–2). Sinus tachycardia is part of the organism's natural reaction to the need for increased oxygen delivery. To the extent that it is a compensatory mechanism, it represents a healthy response to ischemia, exercise, and tissue hypoxia.

Sympathomimetic agents such as *dopamine* and *dobutamine* may produce *positive chronotropic* side effects. Similarly, by blocking parasympathetic activity, *atropine* can also cause an increase in sinus node impulse formation.

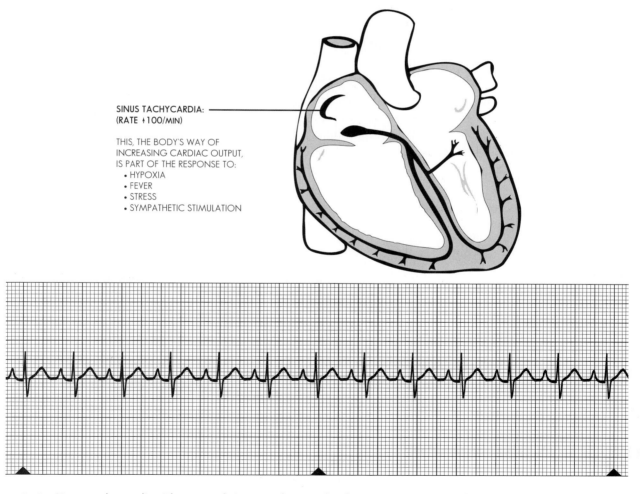

SINUS TACHYCARDIA:
(RATE ∤100/MIN)

THIS, THE BODY'S WAY OF
INCREASING CARDIAC OUTPUT,
IS PART OF THE RESPONSE TO:
• HYPOXIA
• FEVER
• STRESS
• SYMPATHETIC STIMULATION

Figure 8–2. Sinus tachycardia. The rate of sinus node impulse formation is greater than 100/min. The rate in this example is 125/min.

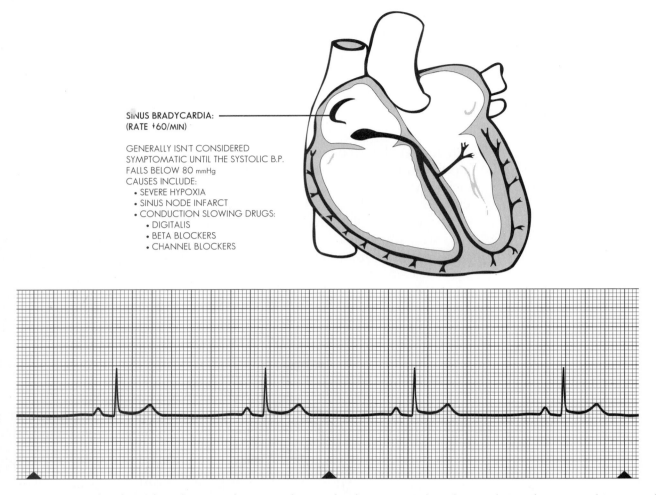

SINUS BRADYCARDIA:
(RATE ↓60/MIN)

GENERALLY ISN'T CONSIDERED
SYMPTOMATIC UNTIL THE SYSTOLIC B.P.
FALLS BELOW 80 mmHg
CAUSES INCLUDE:
• SEVERE HYPOXIA
• SINUS NODE INFARCT
• CONDUCTION SLOWING DRUGS:
    • DIGITALIS
    • BETA BLOCKERS
    • CHANNEL BLOCKERS

Figure 8–3. Sinus bradycardia. The rate of sinus node impulse formation is less than 60/min. The rate in this example is 40/min.

Sinus Bradycardia

When the rate of sinus node impulse formation falls below 60/min, the ECG is called *sinus bradycardia*. As Figure 8–3 indicates, this arrhythmia can result from sinus node ischemia such as occurs with infarct and *severe* hypoxia. It can also be the result of drugs such as the *beta* and *calcium channel blockers*, which slow the rate of impulse formation and conduction.

In the context of ACLS, sinus bradycardia generally does not require treatment until it results in a systolic blood pressure less than 80 mm Hg. Such patients are said to be *hemodynamically unstable*.

CONDUCTION DISTURBANCES

Starting at the sinus node, the conduction system is designed to rapidly deliver action potentials to the Purkinje fibers. ECG signs that this is taking place include:

- PR interval less than 0.20 second.
- Conduction of all P waves.
- QRS complex that is not wider than 0.12 second.

A conduction disturbance is defined as a block or a delay in the journey of the action potential through the conduction system. Of the many that have been described, there are *three patterns* with which the ACLS provider must be familiar.

Unilateral Bundle Branch Block

The interpretation of bundle branch blocks (Figure 8–4) is beyond the scope of an essential ACLS provider course. In general, it is not possible to evaluate the significance *or* the location of this form of block without a 12-lead ECG. The seriousness of bundle branch blocks is essentially that of their underlying causative lesion. That is, if the block is the result of a large infarct, then morbidity would be substantial. The converse is also true.

Bifurcating at the distal end of the His bundle, the right and left bundle branches provide each ventricle with its own electrical circuit. The result is that both chambers fire at *exactly* the same time. Thus, the R wave seen on the normal ECG is actually a *summation* of separate right and left ventricular R waves.

Bundle branch blocks are almost always the result of injury/infarct involving these electrical tracts. Because the normal conduction route is blocked, the action potential must be *rerouted* through slower conducting working cells. This causes the ventricles to discharge asynchronously.

On the ECG this asynchrony is represented by the presence of *two* R waves—an R wave for the unblocked chamber and an R′ wave representing the blocked one.

Therefore, irrespective of which branch is blocked, the R′ wave always occurs *after* the R wave. As can be noted in Figure 8–4, the result is a broad *M-shaped* complex that can be either above or below the isoelectric line.

Nodal AV Block Pattern Associated With First-degree and Second-degree Type I AV Blocks

As illustrated in Figures 8–5, 8–6, and 8–7, when conduction delay occurs in or just below the AV node, the following relationships usually coexist.

- First- and second-degree type I AV blocks are typically seen.
- The disturbance is usually the result of drugs, *not* an infarct. Negative dromotropic agents like *digitalis* and the *beta* and *calcium channel blockers* are frequently implicated.
- The QRS complex is generally within normal limits. This is because the impulse is conducted normally through the ventricles.
- Patients are usually stable hemodynamically. With normal ventricular conduction and few dropped beats, it is rare for these arrhythmias to be the cause of hypotension.

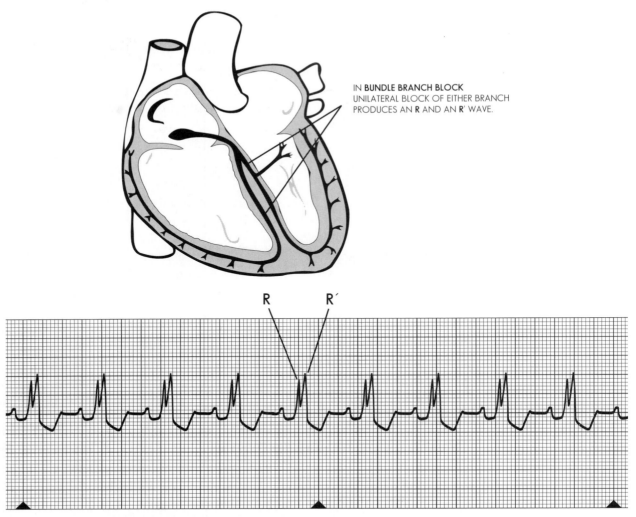

IN **BUNDLE BRANCH BLOCK**
UNILATERAL BLOCK OF EITHER BRANCH
PRODUCES AN **R** AND AN **R'** WAVE.

Figure 8–4. Bundle branch block. With unilateral bundle branch block, the ventricles fire asynchronously resulting in an M-shaped complex with R and R' waves.

- Patients generally do *not* require a pacemaker. Pharmacologic therapy and monitoring are usually all that are required.

Infranodal AV Block Pattern Associated With Second-degree Type II and Third-degree AV Blocks

As illustrated in Figures 8–8, 8–9, and 8–10, when a conduction disturbance occurs at the bundle branch level, the following relationships are typically seen:

- Third-degree or second-degree type II AV block are characteristic.
- The disturbance is usually the result of an ischemic event. As such, the prognosis is considerably poorer than is the case in nodal AV blocks.
- When block occurs below the bundle of His, the QRS tends to be wide.

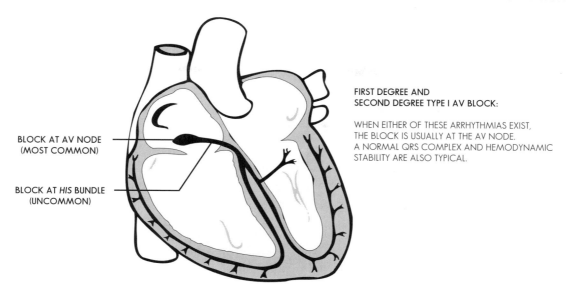

BLOCK AT AV NODE
(MOST COMMON)

BLOCK AT *HIS* BUNDLE
(UNCOMMON)

**FIRST DEGREE AND
SECOND DEGREE TYPE I AV BLOCK:**

WHEN EITHER OF THESE ARRHYTHMIAS EXIST,
THE BLOCK IS USUALLY AT THE AV NODE.
A NORMAL QRS COMPLEX AND HEMODYNAMIC
STABILITY ARE ALSO TYPICAL.

Figure 8–5. *Nodal* block pattern for first- and second-degree type I AV blocks. When conduction delay is in or near the AV node, these two arrhythmias typically result. Because the bundle branches are not involved, the resulting QRS complex is normal.

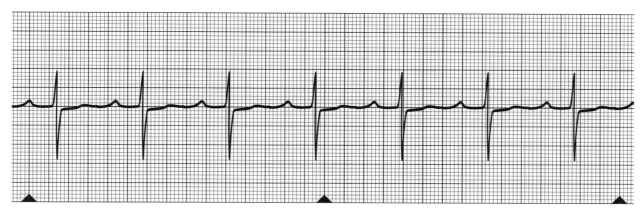

Figure 8–6. First-degree AV block with a PR interval of approximately 0.30 second. The underlying sinus rhythm has a rate of 70/min.

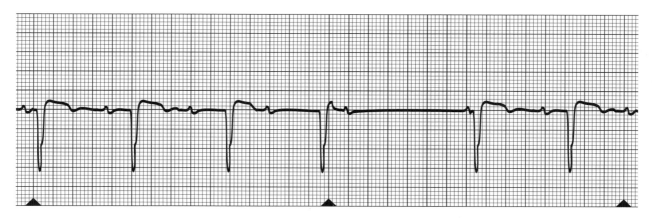

Figure 8–7. Second-degree type I AV block. The criteria for this arrhythmia is sudden dropping of a P wave following gradual widening of the PR interval. In this case the fifth P wave is nonconducted.

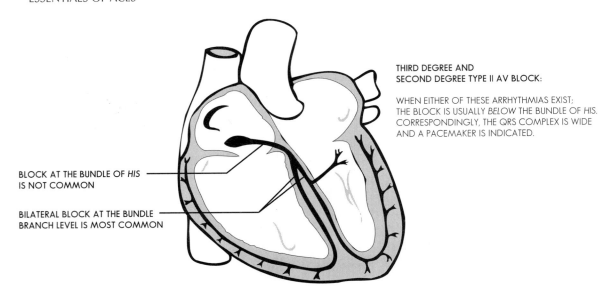

THIRD DEGREE AND
SECOND DEGREE TYPE II AV BLOCK:

WHEN EITHER OF THESE ARRHYTHMIAS EXIST;
THE BLOCK IS USUALLY *BELOW* THE BUNDLE OF *HIS*.
CORRESPONDINGLY, THE QRS COMPLEX IS WIDE
AND A PACEMAKER IS INDICATED.

BLOCK AT THE BUNDLE OF *HIS*
IS NOT COMMON

BILATERAL BLOCK AT THE BUNDLE
BRANCH LEVEL IS MOST COMMON

Figure 8–8. *Infranodal* pattern for third-degree and second-degree type II AV blocks. When the block is at the bundle branch level, anterioseptal MI is often a cause and the prognosis is less favorable.

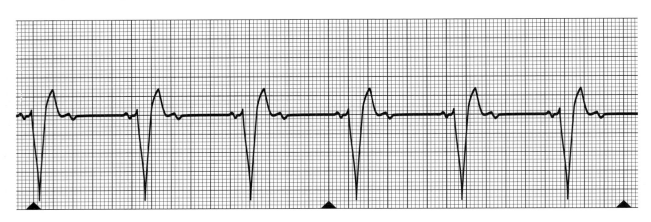

Figure 8–9. Second-degree type II. The criteria for this arrhythmia is sudden dropping of a P wave without widening of the PR interval. In this case, every other beat is dropped.

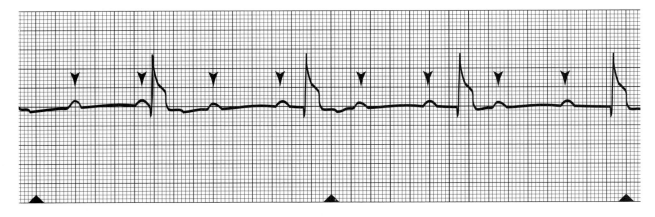

Figure 8–10. Third-degree AV block. Called complete heart block because all P waves are nonconducted. Classically, the sinus node continues to generate impulses at a rate of 60 to 100. At the same time, broad ventricular escape beats are generated at a rate of about 40/min.

- Patients are often hemodynamically unstable. Second-degree type II frequently progresses to third-degree block. Because *all* beats are blocked in the latter instance, systolic blood pressures less than 80 mm Hg are common.
- Patients generally require a pacemaker. A *transvenous* pacemaker is usually required. *Transcutaneous* pacemakers are to be used as a temporizing device until then.

ECTOPIC IMPULSE FORMATION

Just as early defibrillation is the cornerstone of ACLS, the concept of *ectopy* is integral to the discipline of electrocardiology. The word ectopic literally means *originating from an abnormal place*. In cardiology, the term ectopy is used to describe action potentials that originate outside the sinus node.

There are two important mechanisms whereby ectopic impulses may usurp the sinus nodes role as pacemaker of the heart.

Escape Ectopy

Only electrical system cells possess the property of automaticity. Anatomically inferior to the sinus node, distinct groups of pacemaker cells exist. Their function is to "back up" the sinus node should it pause or should impulses not occur.

Clinically, the most important groups of escape pacemaker cells are the ones located in junctional tissues and in the ventricular conduction system.

Junctional Escape Pacemakers

Figure 8–11 illustrates junctional escape pacemakers. The so-called junctional tissues include the AV node, and the bundle of His.

These cells have an inherent or back-up rate of 40 to 60/min. Thus, if there is an interval of time during which the sinus node pauses or doesn't issue an impulse, the junctional tissues will initiate an escape beat. An example of *junctional escape ectopy* appears in Figure 8–12.

In Figure 8–12, note that after a sinus pause of almost 2 seconds, a junctional escape pacemaker fires, discharging the ventricles. Also note that the junctional P wave is inverted. Junctional P waves are inverted because their impulses must undergo *retrograde* conduction to discharge the atria.

As Figure 8–13 illustrates, inverted junctional P waves can precede *or* be hidden within the QRS. Escape impulses of *low* junctional origin may even have to travel farther to discharge the atria than they do to reach the ventricles. In this instance, the inverted P wave occurs *after* the QRS.

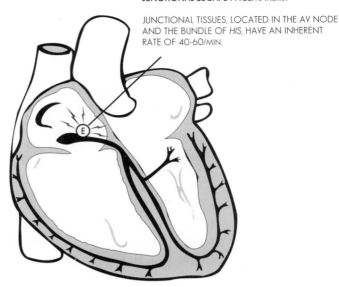

JUNCTIONAL ESCAPE PACEMAKERS:

JUNCTIONAL TISSUES, LOCATED IN THE AV NODE AND THE BUNDLE OF *HIS*, HAVE AN INHERENT RATE OF 40-60/MIN.

Figure 8–11. Illustration of junctional escape pacemakers.

Ventricular Escape Pacemakers

Figure 8–14 illustrates ventricular escape pacemakers. These cells are located in the Purkinje fibers and probably in the bundle branches. Their inherent or escape rate is 40/min or less. Thus, if an impulse from the sinus or the junctional pacemakers does not reach the ventricles in approximately 1.5 seconds (equivalent to a rate of 40/min or less), a ventricular escape pacemaker should fire. Figure 8–15 shows a ventricular escape beat occurring in a patient with sinus bradycardia.

Should complete *supraventricular asystole* occur, there would be no P waves. In this case the ventricles must rely on escape pacemakers with their ideoventricular rate of less than 40/min. This is illustrated in Figure 8–16.

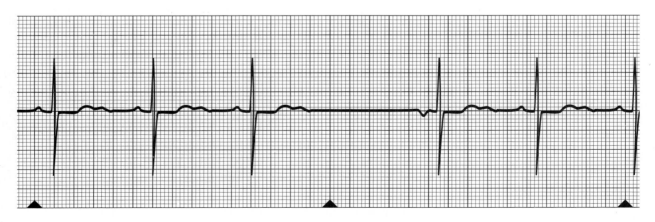

Figure 8–12. Junctional escape ectopy. Please note the presence of sinus pause followed by an inverted junctional P wave which discharges the ventricles. The dominant rhythm has a rate of 60/min. U waves can also be noted after each T wave.

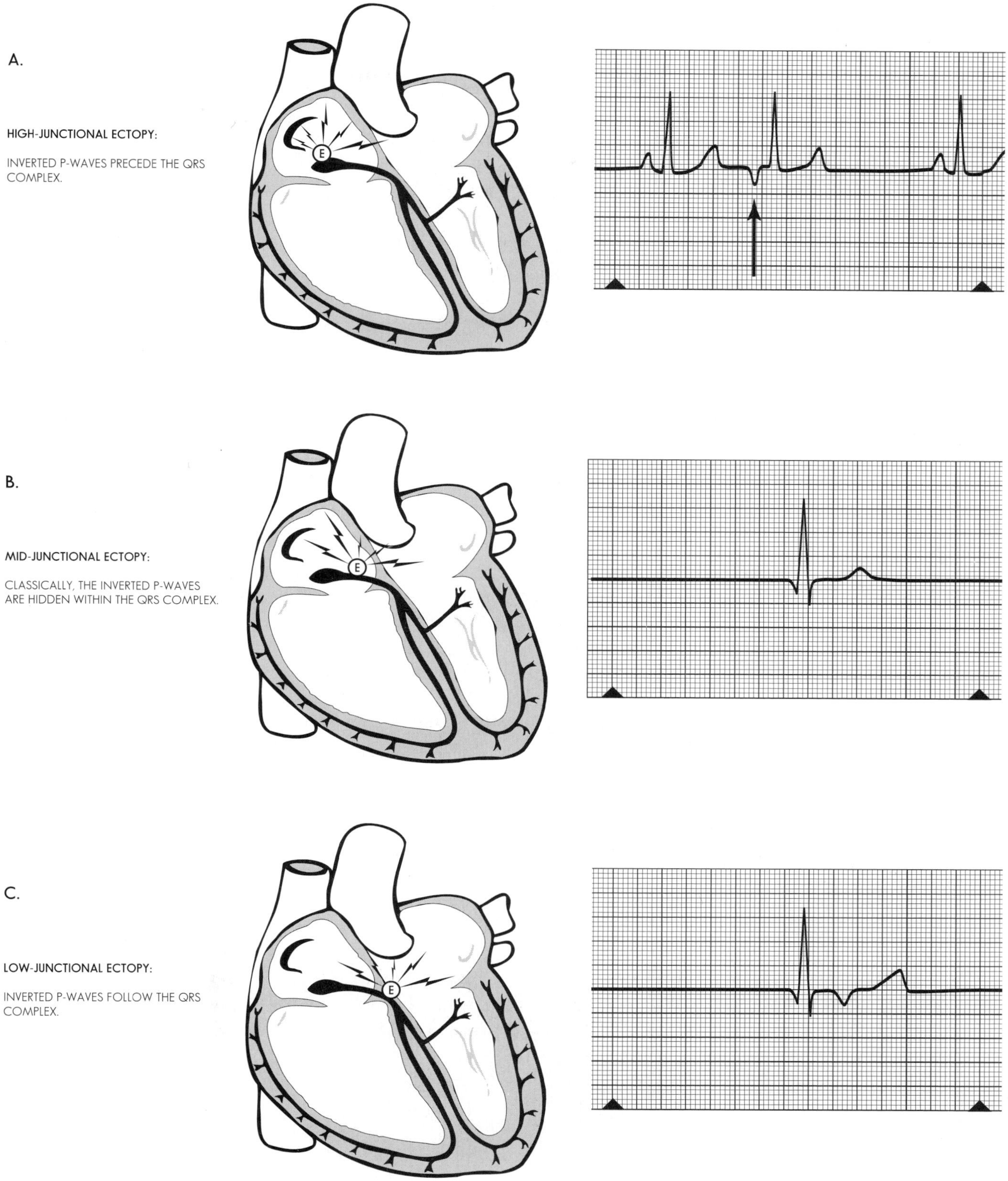

A.

HIGH-JUNCTIONAL ECTOPY:

INVERTED P-WAVES PRECEDE THE QRS COMPLEX.

B.

MID-JUNCTIONAL ECTOPY:

CLASSICALLY, THE INVERTED P-WAVES ARE HIDDEN WITHIN THE QRS COMPLEX.

C.

LOW-JUNCTIONAL ECTOPY:

INVERTED P-WAVES FOLLOW THE QRS COMPLEX.

Figure 8–13. Relationship between the site of origin of junctional ectopy and the position of the junctional P in relation to the QRS. The remarkable phenomenon of the P wave occurring after the QRS complex is illustrated.

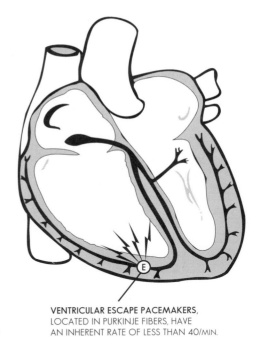

Figure 8–14. Illustration of ventricular escape pacemakers.

VENTRICULAR ESCAPE PACEMAKERS,
LOCATED IN PURKINJE FIBERS, HAVE
AN INHERENT RATE OF LESS THAN 40/MIN.

Note the width of the escape complexes in Figures 8–15 and 8–16. This is typical of ventricular ectopy. Even though the pacemaker cells are located in electrical system cells, the impulse must be conducted through myocardial working cells. These cells are poor conductors; hence, ventricular depolarization takes longer than normal.

Finally, consider third-degree AV block discussed earlier in this chapter. It is called complete heart block because *all* supraventricular impulses (P waves) are *completely* blocked. Once again, the ventricles must rely on their ideoventricular escape rate of 40/min or less. Third-degree AV block is shown again in Figure 8–17.

Perhaps it can be seen that from a clinical standpoint, the ECGs in Figures 8–16 and 8–17 are very similar. That is, since cardiac output and

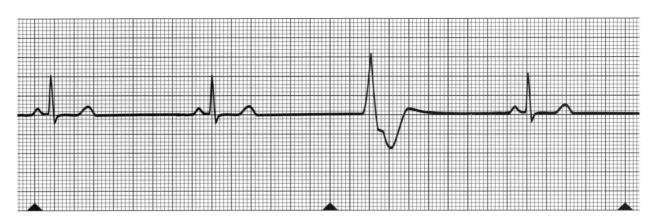

Figure 8–15. Ventricular escape beat. Note the wide complex signifying its conduction outside the bundle branch system.

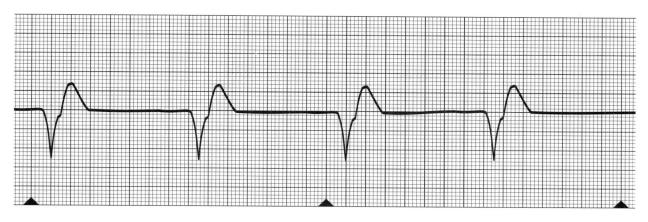

Figure 8–16. Supraventricular asystole with a ventricular escape rhythm.

blood pressure are dependent on broad bradycardic escape complexes these two arrhythmias would probably result in hemodynamic instability.

Premature Ectopy

Of the mechanisms that cause arrhythmias, premature ectopy is most important to the ACLS provider. This is because it is both extremely common and potentially lethal.

It occurs when an irritable focus of cells in either the atria or the ventricles generates an action potential *before* the arrival of the next regular impulse from the sinus node. Premature impulses may be isolated and infrequent or they may occur many times per second, as is the case with ventricular fibrillation.

Table 8–1 shows the relationship between these important arrhythmias and the number of ectopic impulses per minute necessary to cause each. In other words, the electrocardiographic appearance of a patient's cardiac rhythm depends on the rate of ectopic impulse formation.

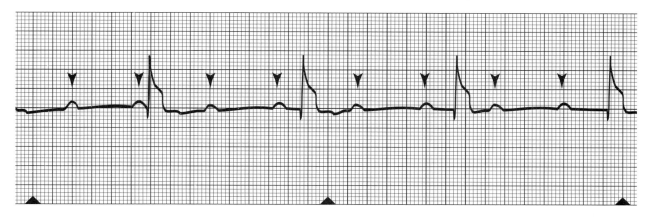

Figure 8–17. Third-degree or complete heart block. None of the P waves are conducted despite appearing on the ECG. The QRS complexes are due to ventricular escape ectopy.

TABLE 8–1. FREQUENCY OF ECTOPIC IMPULSE FORMATION AND SPECIFIC ARRHYTHMIA FORMATION

ATRIAL ARRHYTHMIAS	TYPICAL # ECTOPICS/min.	VENTRICULAR ARRHYTHMIAS	TYPICAL # ECTOPICS/min.
Infrequent PACs	↓ 6	Infrequent PVCs	↓ 6
Frequent PACs	↑ 6	Frequent PVCs	↑ 6
Paroxysmal supraventricular tachycardia (PSVT)	140–220	Ventricular tachycardia (VT)	100–220
Atrial flutter	220–350	Ventricular fibrillation (VF)	220–350
Atrial fibrillation	350–600		

Thus, if an irritable atrial ectopic focus fires 300 times per minute, the ECG will usually meet criteria for atrial flutter. If the focus subsequently begins firing at a rate of 500/min, the ECG will assume the appearance of atrial fibrillation.

There are three additional points that the ACLS provider must understand regarding the clinical significance of arrhythmias resulting from ectopic impulse formation.

- Ventricular ectopy is more serious than atrial ectopy. For example, atrial fibrillation, with its 350 to 600 ectopic per minute, typically results in a 10 to 20% reduction in cardiac output. While often serious enough to precipitate congestive heart failure, it does not compare to ventricular fibrillation. Here the cardiac output ceases, causing clinical death.
- In the first few hours post-AMI, ventricular fibrillation is usually a *precipitous* event. It often develops without any electrocardiographic warning signs such as progressively frequent PVCs.
- Once several hours have passed following AMI, premonitory signs to ventricular fibrillation are common. Frequent and multifocal PVCs, as well as runs of ventricular tachycardia, often forewarn VF/VT and cardiac arrest.

Mechanisms Responsible for Premature Ectopy

There are two important mechanisms responsible for premature ectopy.

Accelerated Automaticity. Pacemaker cells in junctional tissues and in ventricular conductive tissues have been described. These pacemaker cells, especially when adjacent to an area of infarct or injury, can speed their rates dramatically. This accelerated automaticity has been related to abnormalities in slow channel activity.

In any case, when these disturbed cells generate an action potential that is early for the dominant rhythm, the result is a premature contraction. Correspondingly, when highly irritated, these cells can generate hundreds of impulses per minute and cause sudden arrhythmic death.

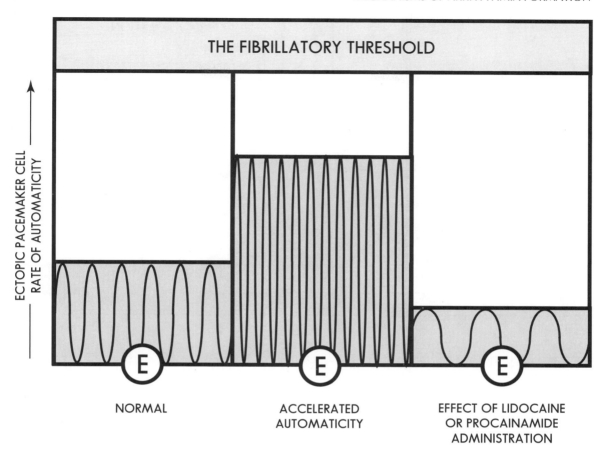

Figure 8–18. Illustration showing the effect of ischemia and antiarrhythmic drugs on the fibrillatory threshold.

Figure 8–18 illustrates accelerated automaticity and introduces the concept of the fibrillatory threshold. This is the difference between the existing rate of pacemaker cell activity and the rate that would be necessary to generate fibrillation.

The drawing in Figure 8–18 illustrates how myocardial ischemia is felt to narrow this threshold. It also shows how administration of antiarrhythmic drugs can act to suppress ectopy.

Major antiarrhythmic drugs such as lidocaine and procainamide are felt to decrease the rate of automaticity of ectopic pacemakers.

Re-entry. The other mechanism that plays a role in premature ectopy is activation of *re-entry* pathways. Cardiologists describe many accessory or alternate conduction routes which are beyond the scope of a basic ACLS course. Re-entry, however, is a mechanism that plays a role in the formation of common atrial and ventricular arrhythmias. For the most part, re-entry circuits amplify the effect of ectopy.

Re-entry allows an ectopic potential to be conducted around an electrical loop at a very rapid rate. Re-entry pathways play a considerable role in PSVT, atrial flutter, and atrial fibrillation. They can also precipitate ventricular tachycardia.

As Figure 8–19 theorizes, a re-entry loop can be established when a

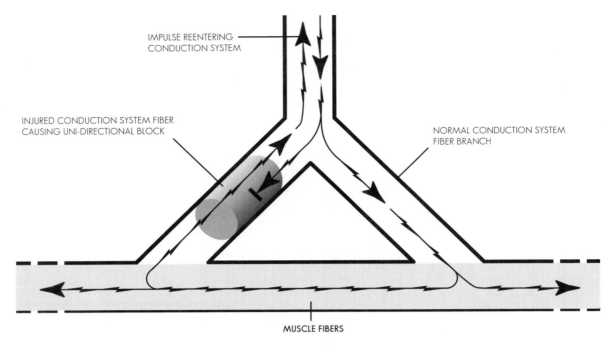

Figure 8–19. Postulated mechanism for creation of a re-entry loop. Rapid discharge of myocardial cells is a known result.

Purkinje fiber becomes injured, causing *unidirectional block*. This permits retrograde conduction, allowing the impulse to *re-enter* the electrical system. This establishes a circuit around which the impulse can travel very quickly.

ARRHYTHMIAS RESULTING FROM PREMATURE ECTOPY

Many of the arrhythmias of concern to the ACLS provider are caused by premature ectopy. These will be discussed below.

Premature Atrial Contractions

As illustrated in Figure 8–20, premature atrial complexes are the result of ectopic pacemakers located in the atria. The sixth P wave, marked by the arrow, has a different morphology or shape reflecting its origin and conduction outside normal pathways.

Note that the sum of the two previous R–R intervals is 0.68 + 0.68 or 1.36 second, whereas the sum of the premature R–R and the *following* R–R is 1.04 second (0.36 + 0.68). This is referred to as an *incomplete compensatory pause* and is typical of PACs. The reason for the incomplete pause is that the ectopic focus is located in the atria. Thus, when it fires, it also depolarizes the sinus node. This acts to "reset" the sinus node's internal clock. The next sinus P wave then occurs earlier than had the PAC not been formed.

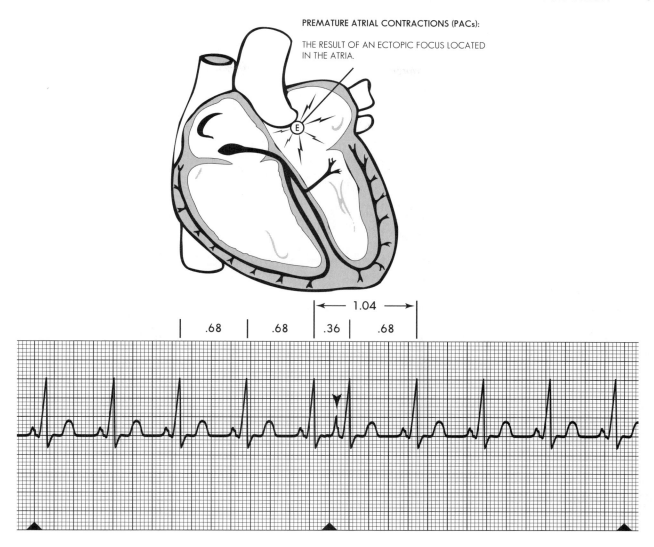

PREMATURE ATRIAL CONTRACTIONS (PACs):

THE RESULT OF AN ECTOPIC FOCUS LOCATED IN THE ATRIA.

Figure 8–20. Premature atrial contraction. Note that the premature beat is early for the dominant rhythm, has a different P wave morphology (see arrow), and is followed by an incomplete compensatory pause.

Paroxysmal Supraventricular Tachycardia

As illustrated in Figure 8–21, paroxysmal supraventricular tachycardia is the result of atrial ectopy *and* a re-entry circuit that involves the AV node. Typically the rate is between 140 and 220/min. PSVT is a sustained run of PACs that classically has an abrupt onset, hence the term paroxysmal. Because the pathology involves the AV node, it can often be terminated by vagal maneuvers.

Atrial Flutter

As illustrated in Figure 8–22 atrial flutter is the result of atrial ectopy and a re-entry loop *not* involving the AV node, this arrhythmia is characterized

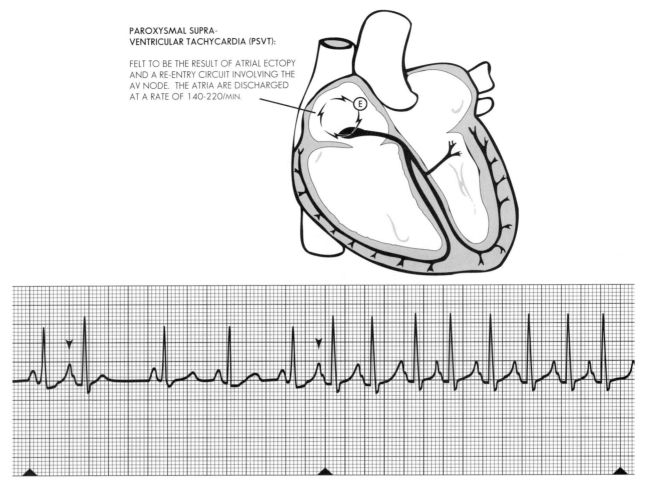

PAROXYSMAL SUPRA-
VENTRICULAR TACHYCARDIA (PSVT):

FELT TO BE THE RESULT OF ATRIAL ECTOPY
AND A RE-ENTRY CIRCUIT INVOLVING THE
AV NODE. THE ATRIA ARE DISCHARGED
AT A RATE OF 140-220/MIN.

Figure 8–21. Paroxysmal supraventricular tachycardia. The second PAC (see arrow) triggers a run of PSVT.

by atrial P waves that resemble saw teeth. It is surprising how often the atrial rate is around 300 per minute. It is also remarkable that the AV node is able to block a majority of these ectopics on an essentially regular basis. Often this mechanism protects against excessive ventricular rates and congestive heart failure (CHF).

Atrial Fibrillation

As illustrated in Figure 8–23, atrial fibrillation results when multiple ectopics and re-entry loops cause the atria to be discharged at rates of 350 to 600/min. Overwhelmed by this *circus movement*, the AV node loses its protective ability to block ectopy on a regular basis.

The result is that the ventricles become discharged on an irregular basis (Figure 8–23). Untreated, ventricular rates often approach 200/min, and congestive heart failure (CHF) is common. Because atrial ectopy is occurring up to ten times per second, the electrocardiographic activity recorded

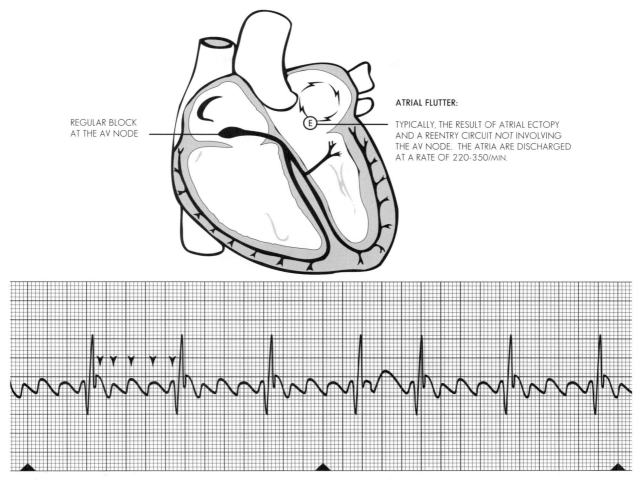

REGULAR BLOCK
AT THE AV NODE

ATRIAL FLUTTER:

TYPICALLY, THE RESULT OF ATRIAL ECTOPY
AND A REENTRY CIRCUIT NOT INVOLVING
THE AV NODE. THE ATRIA ARE DISCHARGED
AT A RATE OF 220-350/MIN.

Figure 8–22. Atrial flutter with 5:1 block. Saw tooth or flutter waves, indicated by arrows, represent atrial ectopic P waves. Every fifth F wave is conducted except between fourth and fifth complex where the conduction ratio is 3:1.

between R waves is chaotic and described as being *fibrillatory* in appearance. Consequently, discernible P waves are *not* visible.

Premature Ventricular Contractions

As illustrated in Figure 8–24 premature ventricular contractions are the result of an irritable ectopic focus located in the ventricles. ECG criteria for PVCs include:

- Early appearance for the dominant rhythm. Thus, the premature R wave occurs just 0.40 second after the last sinus R wave.
- Bizarre appearance. Because they are generated from ectopic locations, impulses are conducted slowly through myocardial working cells.
- A *complete compensatory pause.* Because the ectopic focus is located in the ventricles, the sinus node is *not* depolarized as is the

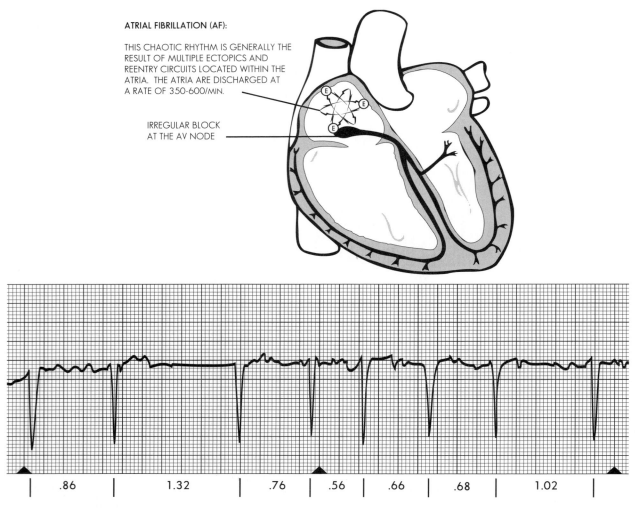

ATRIAL FIBRILLATION (AF):

THIS CHAOTIC RHYTHM IS GENERALLY THE
RESULT OF MULTIPLE ECTOPICS AND
REENTRY CIRCUITS LOCATED WITHIN THE
ATRIA. THE ATRIA ARE DISCHARGED AT
A RATE OF 350-600/MIN.

IRREGULAR BLOCK
AT THE AV NODE

| .86 | 1.32 | .76 | .56 | .66 | .68 | 1.02 |

Figure 8–23. Atrial fibrillation is an irregular irregularity. Its two major characteristics are (1) an irregular R–R interval, and (2) fibrillatory line (between R waves) without discernible P waves.

case with PACs. Thus, the internal clock of the sinus node is not disturbed and the next PQRST sequence occurs right on schedule.

Ventricular Tachycardia (VT)

As illustrated in Figure 8–25, ventricular tachycardia is usually regular in appearance but occasionally may be polymorphic. It is the result of ventricular ectopic foci firing at a rate of 100–220 times per minute.

P waves are generally obscured by broad ventricular ectopic complexes. If not treated promptly, patients rapidly become unstable.

Pulselessness tends to develop as ventricular rates exceed 200/min. At this point, this arrhythmia must be treated with defibrillation according to the VF/VT algorithm.

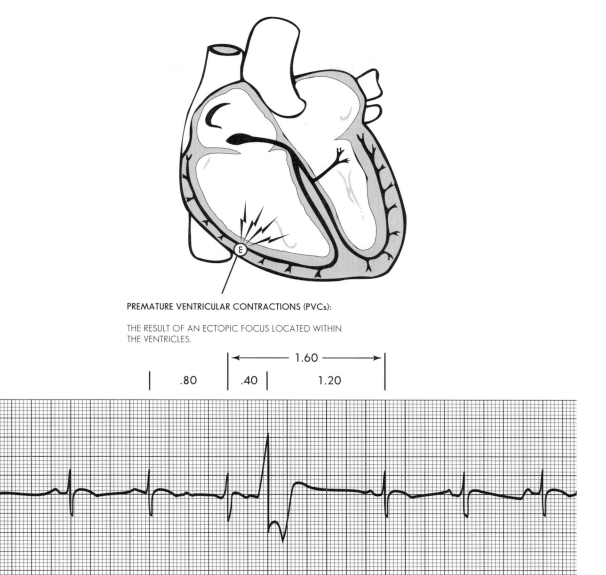

PREMATURE VENTRICULAR CONTRACTIONS (PVCs):

THE RESULT OF AN ECTOPIC FOCUS LOCATED WITHIN
THE VENTRICLES.

Figure 8–24. A single premature ventricular contraction. Note the typical complete compensatory pause.

Ventricular Fibrillation

As illustrated in Figure 8–26, ventricular fibrillation is the result of multiple ventricular ectopic foci firing at rates between 220 to 350 times per minute. The result is electrical chaos as depolarization and repolarization occur simultaneously throughout the ventricular muscle mass. Not surprisingly this arrhythmia produces no stroke volume or cardiac output. *Clinical death*, as manifested by pulselessness and unconsciousness, occurs suddenly.

Following AMI between 80 and 90% of cases of cardiac arrest are due to VF. If treated within two minutes with defibrillation, survival rates often exceed 80%.

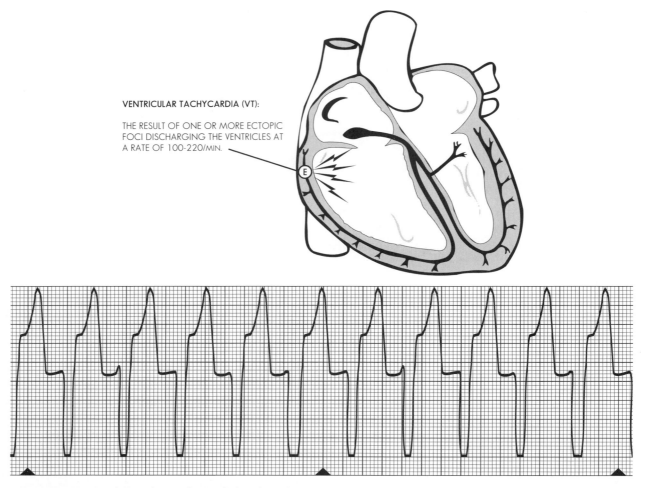

VENTRICULAR TACHYCARDIA (VT):

THE RESULT OF ONE OR MORE ECTOPIC FOCI DISCHARGING THE VENTRICLES AT A RATE OF 100-220/MIN.

Figure 8–25. Ventricular tachycardia is defined as three or more PVCs in a row. Runs lasting more that 30 seconds are called sustained VT.

If defibrillation is delayed ten minutes from the onset of VF, survival rates fall below 10%.

That is why the single most important goal of ACLS is to provide early defibrillation to victims of cardiac arrest.

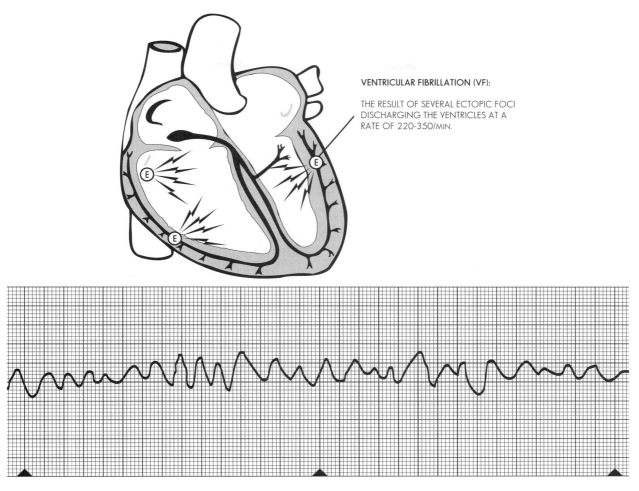

VENTRICULAR FIBRILLATION (VF):

THE RESULT OF SEVERAL ECTOPIC FOCI DISCHARGING THE VENTRICLES AT A RATE OF 220-350/MIN.

Figure 8–26. Ventricular fibrillation. Heralded by pulselessness and unconsciousness, this catastrophic arrhythmia is responsible for 80 to 90% of cases of non-traumatic adult cardiac arrest.

BIBLIOGRAPHY

1. American Heart Association, Emergency Cardiac Care Committee and Subcommittees. Guidelines for cardiopulmonary resuscitation and emergency cardiac care. JAMA 1992;268:2171–2295

2. American Heart Association. Textbook of advanced cardiac life support. Dallas, TX: American Heart Association, 1994

3. American Heart Association. Instructor's manual for advanced cardiac life support. Dallas, TX: American Heart Association, 1994

4. Meltzer LE, Pinneo R, and Kitchell JR. *Intensive Coronary Care*, 4th ed. Norwalk CT: Appleton & Lange, 1983.

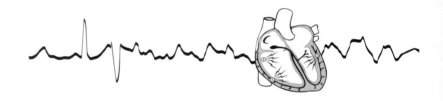

9. Therapeutic Agents of the ACLS Algorithms

OUTLINE

Essential ACLS Curricula

Glossary of Pharmacologic Terms

Agents Recommended in the Cardiac Arrest Algorithms
- Oxygen
- IV fluids
- Epinephrine
- Atropine
- Sodium bicarbonate

Agents Recommended in the Acute Myocardial Infarction Algorithm
- Oxygen
- Nitroglycerin
- Morphine
- Aspirin
- Thrombolytic agents
- Heparin
- Beta blockers
- Lidocaine
- Magnesium sulfate
- Percutaneous Transluminal Coronary Angioplasty (PCTA)

Agents of the Acute Pulmonary Edema/Hypotension/Shock Algorithm
- Norepinephrine
- Dopamine
- Dobutamine
- Nitroglycerin and Nitroprusside
- Furosemide

Agents of the VF/VT and Tachycardia Algorithms
- Lidocaine
- Procainamide
- Bretylium
- Magnesium sulfate
- Vagal maneuvers
- Adenosine
- Verapamil
- Diltiazem
- Beta blockers

Agents Recommended in the Bradycardia Algorithm
- Atropine
- Transcutaneous Pacing
- Dopamine and Epinephrine
- Isoproterenol

ESSENTIAL ACLS CURRICULA

The current AHA *Instructor's Manual for ACLS* states that for therapeutic modalities and pharmacologic agents identified as essential for ACLS courses, participants must know:

- Mechanisms of action (*why* an agent is used).
- Indications relevant to ACLS (*when* to use a given agent).
- The dosage for each indication (*how* the drug is used).
- The hazards and precautions associated with each modality (*what* to watch out for).

These instructor guidelines state that the following agents should be taught as part of an essential ACLS provider course:

- IV fluids
- Oxygen
- Epinephrine
- Lidocaine
- Bretylium
- Magnesium sulfate
- Procainamide
- Sodium bicarbonate
- Atropine
- Dopamine
- Isoproterenol
- Vagal maneuvers (used as a drug)
- Adenosine
- Verapamil
- Diltiazem
- Beta blockers (atenolol, propranolol, metoprolol, or esmolol)
- Nitroglycerin
- Nitroprusside
- Dobutamine
- Morphine sulfate
- Furosemide
- A thrombolytic agent (the one used in the provider's work setting)

As ACLS course participants are aware, the "blueprints" for administering these drugs and therapeutic agents are the nine essential ACLS algorithms.

Your ACLS course is built around these critical pathways. The nine case-based Performance Stations are structured to evaluate participant understanding of these algorithms.

This review text is designed to assist your mastery of this educational approach. Therefore, the above agents will be discussed in the context of the algorithm(s) that provide guidelines for their use in ACLS.

GLOSSARY OF PHARMACOLOGIC TERMS

Adrenergic: Pertaining to or acting upon the sympathetic nervous system.

Afterload: The vascular pressure and resistance against which the left or right ventricle must eject its stroke volume.

Agonist: A drug or agent that acts upon a specific group of receptor or target cells.

Alpha-1 adrenergic receptors: These are located primarily in vascular smooth muscle. Stimulation results in arterial and/or venous *vasoconstriction*. Alpha-1 adrenergic agonists such as dopamine and norephrinephrine are mainstays in managing heart failure accompanied by hypotension.

Alpha-2 adrenergic receptors: These are located primarily in the pre- and post-synaptic effector sites of vascular and myocardial muscle cells. They regulate stimulation of alpha-1 receptors by limiting the activity of norepinephrine.

Antagonist: A drug or agent that exerts a *blocking* action on a specific group of receptors or target cells.

Beta-1 adrenergic receptors: Located in the myocardium. Stimulation results in positive inotropic, chronotropic, or dromotropic actions.

Beta-2 adrenergic receptors: Located in smooth muscle of the bronchioles and in blood vessels. Stimulation results in *vasodilatation* and *bronchodilatation*.

Cholinergic: Pertaining to or acting upon the parasympathetic nervous system.

Chronotropic effect: A pharmacologic action that results in an increase (positive effect) or a decrease (negative effect) in heart rate.

Dopaminergic receptors: Located in renal and mesenteric blood vessels. Stimulation results in *vasodilatation*.

Dromotropic effect: A pharmacologic action that results in speeding up (positive effect) or slowing down (negative effect) of conduction through the AV node.

Inotropic effect: A pharmacologic action that results in an increase (positive effect) or a decrease (negative effect) in the force or strength of myocardial contraction.

Parasympathetic nervous system: The "conservative and homeostatic" branch of the autonomic nervous system whose actions are mediated by the neurotransmitter acetylcholine. In general, stimulation of the parasympathetic nervous system results in:

- Negative inotropic, chronotropic, and dromotropic myocardial actions
- Bronchoconstriction
- Stimulation of the gastrointestinal system
- Increased salivatory and mucus gland production
- Pupillary constriction

Parasympatholitic action: To therapeutically block the actions of the parasympathetic nervous system.

Parasympathomimetic action: To therapeutically stimulate the actions of the parasympathetic nervous system.

Preload: The filling pressure of the right or left ventricle. The pulmonary wedge pressure (PWP), used clinically to approximate the left heart filling pressure, is characteristically elevated in congestive heart failure (CHF).

Sympathetic nervous system: The "fight or flight" branch of the autonomic nervous system whose actions are mediated by the neurotransmitter norepinephrine. In general, stimulation of the sympathetic nervous system results in:

- Positive inotropic, chronotropic, and dromotropic myocardial actions if beta-1 receptors are stimulated

- Bronchodilitation if beta-2 receptors are stimulated
- Vasoconstriction if alpha-1 receptors are stimulated
- Vasodilitation if beta-2 receptors are stimulated

Sympatholytic action: To therapeutically block the actions of the sympathetic nervous system.

Sympathomimetic action: To therapeutically stimulate the actions of the sympathetic nervous system.

Vasopressor agents: Drugs such as norepinephrine and dopamine that produce arterial and/or venous vasoconstrictions.

AGENTS RECOMMENDED IN THE CARDIAC ARREST ALGORITHMS

Overview

The asystole, PEA, and VF/VT algorithms share the following therapeutic interventions:

- Oxygen
- IV fluids
- Epinephrine
- Atropine
- Sodium bicarbonate

These algorithms are presented in Chapter 10, which is devoted to the lethal arrhythmias. Please review them as necessary.

Oxygen

Mechanisms of Action (Why)

Oxygen is a fundamental therapeutic modality. Wherever possible, patients requiring ACLS should have an arterial oxygen saturation of 97% or greater. Particularly valuable in the ACLS setting is the ability of oxygen to:

- Increase SaO_2 and arterial oxygen content.
- Help prevent metabolic acidosis by increasing the amount of oxygen transported to the tissues.
- Reduce the magnitude and extent of ST segment changes in patients with AMI.

Indications (When)

- Cardiac arrest
- Ischemic chest pain
- Suspected hypoxemia of any cause

Dosage (How)

- 100% oxygen for *cardiac arrest.* Typically, this is administered via a bag–valve–reservoir unit.
- 4 to 6 L/min via nasal cannula for patients in *mild respiratory distress.* This corresponds to about 36 to 44% inspired oxygen.
- 40 to 100% oxygen for patients with *moderate to severe* respiratory distress.

  Simple oxygen masks run at flows of 6 to 10 L/min and deliver 40 to 60% oxygen.

  Partial rebreathing masks run at flows of 8 to 12 L/min and deliver 60 to 80% oxygen.

  Non-rebreathing masks run at flows of 8 to 12 L/min amd deliver 80 to 100% oxygen.

Hazards

Patients with chronic obstructive pulmonary disease may be at risk for oxygen-induced hypoventilation. For these individuals, do not withhold oxygen, monitor, and be prepared to support ventilation.

IV Fluids

Mechanisms of Action (Why)

The guidelines state that *normal saline* or *lactated Ringer's* are preferred infusion fluids during ACLS. Five percent dextrose solutions are considered *merely acceptable.*

Indications (When)

- **Volume expansion.** Hypovolemia is the most common treatable cause of pulseless electrical activity (PEA). Thus, volume expansion is part of the treatment of PEAs. Volume infusion is also indicated in the management of systemic hypotension prior to the administration of vasopressor agents.
- To keep IV lines open for drug administration.

Dosage (How)

- Infusion rates of 10 mL/h are recommended to keep IV lines open.
- If indicated, one or more 250-mL fluid challenges can be given over a short period of time. If the patient's response is not satisfactory, pressor agents can be considered.

- A 20-mL bolus of fluid should be given after each dose of IV medications given during cardiac arrest. The extremity should then be elevated.

Hazards

Routine volume expansion is felt to be potentially hazardous in the cardiac arrest patient. Volume loading performed without indication in these patients can lead to decreased coronary and cerebral perfusion.

Epinephrine

Mechanisms of Action (Why)

Epinephrine is the only class I therapeutic agent for all three manifestations of cardiac arrest. No other agent is associated with higher outcomes. Its primary mechanisms of action are to:

- Increase coronary and cerebral blood flow. Epinephrine has potent alpha-adrenergic stimulating properties. This results in marked increases in peripheral vascular resistance.
- Restore electrical activity in asystole.
- Enhance defibrillation in refractory VF/VT.

Indications (When)

- **Cardiac arrest.** Epinephrine is the *first-line* IV medication in all forms of cardiac arrest.
    VF/VT
    Asystole
    PEA
- **Symptomatic bradycardia.** Here it is recommended after atropine, TCP, and dopamine.

Dosage (How)

- **Cardiac arrest.** *First dose:* 1 mg IV push, may repeat every 3 to 5 minutes. *Alternative regimes for second dose of epinephrine (class IIb):*
    Intermediate: 2 to 5 mg IV push, every 3 to 5 min.
    Escalating: 1 mg, 3 mg, 5 mg IV push, 3 min apart.
    High: 0.1 mg/kg IV push every 3 to 5 min.
- **Endotracheal.** 2.0 to 2.5 mg diluted in 10 mL normal saline (NS) or distilled water.
- **Profound bradycardia.** 2 to 10 µg/min (add 1 mg to 500 mL NS; run at 1 to 5 mL/min).

Hazards

- **Worsening of ischemia.** Epinephrine's positive chronotropic action can increase myocardial oxygen demand.
- **Hypertension.** High doses can produce hypertension. Fortunately, this drug is metabolized quickly.
- **Inactivation in alkaline solutions.** Epinephrine should never be administered in solutions that contain sodium bicarbonate or calcium salts.

Atropine

Mechanisms of Action (Why)

Atropine is a *parasympathetic antagonist*. Its action is to block vagal impulses. This results in sympathetic dominance. In terms of the heart, this means:

- **A positive *chronotropic* effect.** The rate of automaticity of the sinus node is increased.
- **A positive *dromotropic* effect.** Conduction through the AV node is accelerated. Electrocardiographically, this action is manifested in narrowing of the PR interval.

Indications (When)

- **Cardiac arrest due to asystole or bradycardic PEA (class IIb).** Atropine is the *second-line* IV agent. It is used after epinephrine.
- **Symptomatic bradycardias (class I).** It is the *first-line* IV medication for sinus bradycardia, as well as second- and third-degree AV blocks. When these arrhythmias are the result of AMI, atropine is valuable as a temporizing agent until a transcutaneous pacemaker can be placed.

Dosage (How)

- **Asystole or slow PEA.** 1 mg IV push. Repeat every 3 to 5 min (if asystole persists) to maximum dose of 0.04 mg/kg.
- **Symptomatic bradycardia.** 0.5 to 1.0 mg IV every 3 to 5 min as needed; not to exceed total dose of 0.04 mg/kg.
- **Endotracheal dose.** 1 to 2.5 mg diluted in 10 mL NS or distilled water.

Hazards

Because of its positive chronotropic effect, atropine increases myocardial oxygen demand. Thus, it should be used with caution in patients with myocardial ischemia and injury. The JAMA guidelines state that atropine should be used with caution in the following settings:

- Bradycardia due to AMI (class IIb).
- Patients with second-degree type II and third-degree AV blocks with broad QRS complexes (class IIb).

Sodium Bicarbonate

Mechanisms of Action (Why)

Sodium bicarbonate is considered a class III or *harmful* agent in prolonged cardiac arrest when the patient is *not intubated*. It is a class IIb or *possibly helpful* agent in prolonged cardiac arrest when the patient *is intubated*.

The reason for this is that sodium bicarbonate, after buffering lactic or other strong acids, forms carbonic acid, which then dissociates into CO_2 and water. Thus, unless the patient is intubated and being ventilated, sodium bicarbonate administration will actually worsen acidosis.

Well-performed adult CPR consists of 60 chest compressions and 10 to 15 ventilations per minute. The tidal volume for these ventilations should be 10 to 15 mL/kg. This will result in a cardiac output 20 to 30% of normal and mild to moderate hyperventilation.

The marked drop in oxygen tissue delivery causes the cells to shift into anaerobic metabolic pathways. This results in the accumulation of lactic acid and carbon dioxide in the venous blood. Mixed venous blood during CPR has a pH of about 7.15, a $P\bar{v}CO_2$ of approximately 70 mm and a mild base deficit.

With the addition of hyperventilation, excessive carbon dioxide is removed. Thus, the pH of arterial blood during CPR performed with adequate ventilation is slightly alkalotic. The anomaly of venous acidosis existing despite arterial alkalosis has been termed the "*venoarterial paradox*."

In light of this, the JAMA guidelines state that provision of adequate alveolar ventilation during cardiac arrest is the "mainstay" in controlling acid–base balance.

Indications (When)

Sodium bicarbonate is *not* recommended for routine use in patients with cardiac arrest.

The JAMA guidelines state that it be considered only after mainstream interventions such as defibrillation, compressions, intubation, and *more than one* trial of epinephrine.

Specific indications for sodium bicarbonate as listed in the VF/VT, asystole, and PEA algorithms are as follows:

- *Class I* if patient has known pre-existing hyperkalemia.
- *Class IIa* if known pre-existing bicarbonate-responsive acidosis (eg, diabetic ketoacidosis), tricyclic antidepressant overdose, or to alkalinize urine as in aspirin or barbiturate overdose.
- *Class IIb* if intubated and continued long arrest interval; upon return of spontaneous circulation after long arrest interval.
- *Class III* (harmful): for prolonged cardiac arrest and CPR without intubation.

Dosage (How)

- Sodium bicarbonate is given as a 1 mEq/kg IV bolus. Repeat half this dose every 10 minutes thereafter. If readily available, use blood gas analysis to guide administration.

Hazards

- Release of CO_2 and worsening of acidosis.
  HCO_3 combines with the H+ contributed by strong acids to produce the weaker carbonic acid (H_2CO_3).
  Carbonic acid then dissociates into water and carbon dioxide (CO_2) molecules.
  During cardiac arrest, sodium bicarbonate administration can cause carbon dioxide accumulation and unwanted acidosis in myocardial cells, the cerebrospinal fluid (CSF), and the venous circulation.
- Hypernatremia and hyperosmolality.
- Leftward shift in the oxyhemoglobin dissociation curve.
- Inactivation of catecholamines and calcium salts when administered concurrently.

AGENTS RECOMMENDED IN THE ACUTE MYOCARDIAL INFARCTION ALGORITHM

Overview

Every year in the United States, several million victims with chest pain and other symptoms of AMI call 911 seeking rapid access to emergency care.

The acute myocardial infarction algorithm (Figure 9–1) offers recommendations for the management of the patient with possible AMI. These guidelines outline responsibilities in the domain of the community, the emergency medical service (EMS) system, and the emergency department.

The emphasis of this team approach is to employ thrombolytic therapy as quickly as possible if indicated. Specific responsibilities are discussed below.

Acute Myocardial Infarction Algorithm
Recommendations for early management of patients with chest pain and possible AMI

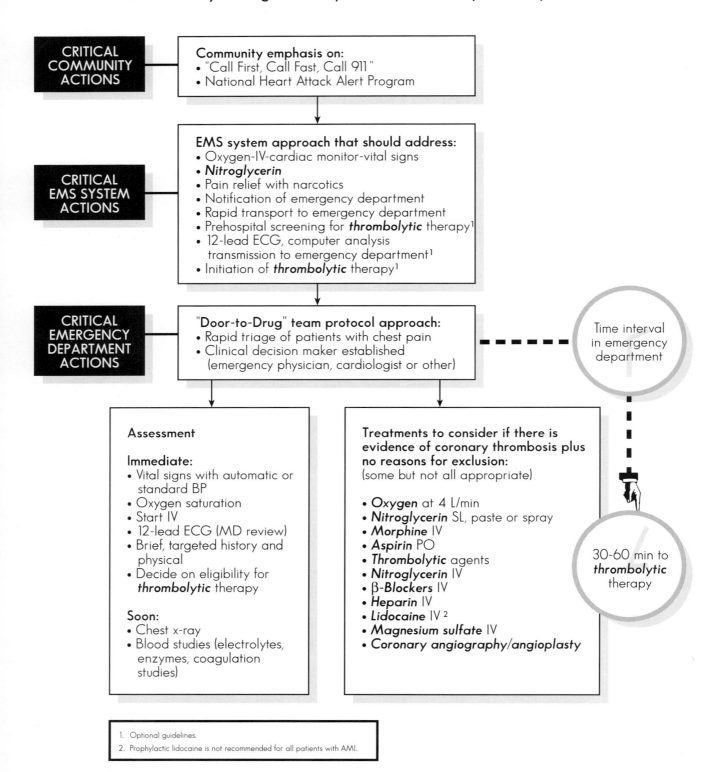

CRITICAL COMMUNITY ACTIONS

Community emphasis on:
• "Call First, Call Fast, Call 911"
• National Heart Attack Alert Program

CRITICAL EMS SYSTEM ACTIONS

EMS system approach that should address:
• Oxygen-IV-cardiac monitor-vital signs
• *Nitroglycerin*
• Pain relief with narcotics
• Notification of emergency department
• Rapid transport to emergency department
• Prehospital screening for *thrombolytic* therapy[1]
• 12-lead ECG, computer analysis transmission to emergency department[1]
• Initiation of *thrombolytic* therapy[1]

CRITICAL EMERGENCY DEPARTMENT ACTIONS

"Door-to-Drug" team protocol approach:
• Rapid triage of patients with chest pain
• Clinical decision maker established (emergency physician, cardiologist or other)

Time interval in emergency department

Assessment

Immediate:
• Vital signs with automatic or standard BP
• Oxygen saturation
• Start IV
• 12-lead ECG (MD review)
• Brief, targeted history and physical
• Decide on eligibility for *thrombolytic* therapy

Soon:
• Chest x-ray
• Blood studies (electrolytes, enzymes, coagulation studies)

Treatments to consider if there is evidence of coronary thrombosis plus no reasons for exclusion:
(some but not all appropriate)

• *Oxygen* at 4 L/min
• *Nitroglycerin* SL, paste or spray
• *Morphine* IV
• *Aspirin* PO
• *Thrombolytic* agents
• *Nitroglycerin* IV
• β-*Blockers* IV
• *Heparin* IV
• *Lidocaine* IV [2]
• *Magnesium sulfate* IV
• *Coronary angiography/angioplasty*

30-60 min to *thrombolytic* therapy

1. Optional guidelines.
2. Prophylactic lidocaine is not recommended for all patients with AMI.

Figure 9–1. The acute myocardial infarction algorithm. This critical pathway is evaluated in Case 6, Acute Myocardial Infarction. (Algorithm copyright 1992, American Medical Association; JAMA, October 28, 1992, pp 2199–2241.)

Community Responsibility

It is the role of the community to emphasize the importance of early entry to the EMS system. The public must be taught that symptoms such as chest pain and shortness of breath are early warning signs that must not be ignored. The average time of 3 to 4 hours from onset of symptoms to seeking of help is not acceptable.

Responsibilities of the EMS System

The EMS system consists of *dispatchers* and paramedic *responders*. These individuals work in concert to assure that trained personnel and life-support equipment reaches the victim in an acceptable amount of time. The goal of the American Heart Association is to provide CPR and ACLS in less than 4 minutes. In both densely and sparsely populated (urban and rural) areas, this goal remains a formidable challenge.

As the AMI algorithm indicates, once EMS responders arrive at the scene of a patient with chest pain and possible AMI, responsibilities include *monitoring, providing oxygen, IV access,* and *pain relief.* Stabilized, the patient must be transported to the emergency department as rapidly as possible.

Responsibilities of the Emergency Department

Once the patient arrives in the emergency department, the *"door-to-drug"* interval begins. This is the amount of time that it takes for ER personnel to determine the need for and begin administration of *thrombolytic agents.* As the AMI algorithm indicates, the guidelines recommend that this take no more than 30 to 60 minutes. You will remember from the discussion of myocardial injury in Chapter 7 that the decision to initiate thrombolytic therapy is made upon analysis of ST segment changes on the 12-lead ECG. In general, if ST segment elevation of 1 mm or more is noted in two contiguous leads, the patient is presumed to be *"myocardially infarcting."*

The emergency department should be staffed by specially trained physicians. These individuals must consider a defined group of therapeutic interventions for the patient who presents with signs and symptoms of AMI. These treatments are outlined in Figure 9–1 and discussed in the text that follows.

Oxygen Therapy for Suspected AMI

The patient with signs and symptoms of uncomplicated AMI should receive 4 to 6 L/min oxygen via nasal cannula. This is thought to be the equivalent of 36 to 44% inspired oxygen concentration. Pulse oximetry should be used to titrate oxygen administration so that SaO_2s greater than 97% are achieved.

Nitroglycerin (PO and IV)

Mechanisms of Action (Why)

Used early in the patient with suspected AMI, nitroglycerin has an effect on outcomes and infarct size comparable to that of thrombolytic agents. This old standby achieves its beneficial effects by dilating vascular smooth muscle. It works independently of the autonomic nervous system. Its beneficial effects in the management of AMI stem from the following vascular actions:

- **Dilatation of coronary arteries.** This action often yields dramatic reductions in ischemic pain.
- **Dilatation of both venules and arterioles.** This action helps unload the left ventricle by decreasing venous return and reducing left heart afterload.

Indications (When)

- Acute angina pectoris.
- Suspected AMI *without* hypotension.
- Complicated AMI with systolic blood pressure greater than 100 mm Hg.

Dosage (How)

- **Sublingual.** 0.3 to 0.4 mg repeated every 5 min.
- **Inhaler.** One spray every 5 min.
- **Intravenous dose.** Infuse at 10 to 20 μg/min. Titrate to effect, keeping the systolic BP greater than 90 mm Hg.

Hazards

The main hazard is *hypotension*. The patient should not stand, as syncope may occur. In general, limit drops in systolic BP to 10% in normotensive patients and to 30% in hypertensive patients.

Morphine (IV)

Mechanisms of Action (Why)

Patients who suffer an AMI characterize their pain in the severest of terms. More importantly, the *sympathetic outpouring* that accompanies this pain increases myocardial oxygen demands and systemic vascular resistance. In the setting of AMI, morphine is an extremely valuable agent because it produces the following actions:

- **Relief of anginal pain.** Morphine is a powerful *analgesic*. Given IV, it provides relief from pain and anxiety almost immediately.
- **Increase in venous capacitance.** Morphine dilates venous smooth muscle. This action has been called a *pharmacologic phlebotomy*. It results in a diminishment of the preload to the heart.
- **Acts synergistically with nitroglycerin.**

Indications (When)

- Relief of chest pain and anxiety associated with AMI.
- Relief of pulmonary vascular congestion in patients with acute cardiogenic pulmonary edema. Here it is considered a class IIb agent (possibly helpful) for use *only* if the systolic blood pressure is greater than 90 mm Hg.

Dosage (How)

Morphine is given 1 to 3 mg IV. This dose can be given as often as every 5 minutes to achieve pain relief.

Hazards

- **Respiratory center depression.** Morphine must be used with caution in patients with chronic obstructive pulmonary disease (COPD) and in patients with acute pulmonary edema who are in severe distress.
- **Hypotension.** Morphine should *not* be used in volume-depleted patients or in those with a systolic BP less than 90 mm Hg.
- Reverse with naloxone (0.4 to 0.8 mg IV) if necessary. It is helpful to remember that naloxone can be administered endotracheally.

Aspirin (PO)

Mechanisms of Action (Why)

Aspirin (160 to 325 mg PO) is a class I (definitely helpful) agent that should be given to *all* patients with suspected AMI. This includes those to receive thrombolytic therapy.

Remarkably, when administered alone within 24 hours of an AMI, PO aspirin has produced reductions in mortality almost as large as are seen with the use of thrombolytic agents. Aspirin inhibits the formation of thromboxane A_2. This substance causes platelets to aggregate. Limiting of platelet agglutination has been demonstrated to improve outcomes and reduce nonfatal *reinfarction*.

Indications (When)

Aspirin should be given as soon as possible as standard therapy to all patients with suspected AMI. In most EMS systems, paramedics administer aspirin in the pre-hospital setting.

Dosage (How)

Aspirin is given 160 to 325 mg PO. Flavored chewable children's aspirin contain 160 mg/tablet. Adult tablets contain 325 mg. Higher doses can cancel out beneficial effects.

Hazards

- Aspirin is contraindicated in patients with known hypersensitivity.
- Relative contraindications exist for patients with gastric ulcers and for asthmatic patients.

Thrombolytic Agents

Role in ACLS

Most AMIs are caused by *thrombotic occlusion* of a coronary artery. Typically, a blood clot forms on the jagged surfaces of a coronary artery injured by an atherosclerotic lesion. Thrombolytic agents act to dissolve these clots. Thus, they can actually *reopen* blocked arteries. Not surprisingly, these agents are most effective when given shortly after the onset of AMI. The AMI algorithm (Figure 9–1) reflects this focus. Thus, it indicates that the primary goal of the emergency department team is to administer these agents (if indicated) within 30 to 60 minutes of the patient's arrival in the ER. This process is called the "door-to-drug interval."

Speed is critical if the health care team is to "salvage" injured myocardium. The JAMA guidelines emphasize the concept that for the patient who is myocardially infarcting, "time is muscle."

Figures 9–2 and 9–3 present 12-lead ECG studies performed on a patient who began receiving streptokinase approximately 30 minutes after experiencing sudden severe chest pain. You will note in Figure 9–2 ST segment changes in leads II, III, and aVF which are consistent with an *inferior injury*. Also note the reciprocal ST segment changes in leads V_1, V_2, and V_3.

Figure 9–3 is an ECG recording obtained approximately 30 minutes after administration of streptokinase was begun. Please note the improvement in the ST segment. In addition, conversion from junctional tachycardia to a sinus rhythm is seen.

17:31:47

Rate	103	. Junctional tachycardia, rate 103
PR	101	$ Long R-R interval measured
QRSD	335	. Inferior injury (ACUTE INFARCT)
QT	335	with reciprocal ST depression
QTc	438	. Anterolateral T wave abnormalities
		. . consistent with ischemia
--AXIS--		$ Baseline wander in lead(s) V1, V3, V4, V5, V6
P		
QRS	86	
T	94	

- ABNORMAL ECG -

Absent P waves, rate >= 100DOB:
R-R interval > 140% of normal
ST > .35 mv in II, III, aVFMR:

T waves - .60 mv I, aVL,V2-V6
T > -.60 mv

PRELIMINARY-MD MUST REVIEW

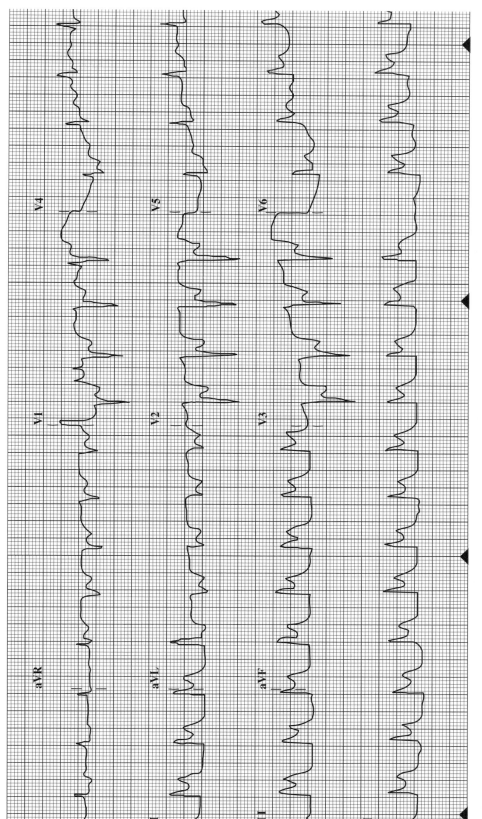

Figure 9–2. 12-lead ECG performed 20 minutes after the onset of crushing substernal chest pain. Note the ST segment abnormalities in leads II, III, aVF, V_1, V_2, and V_3.

18:09:50

Rate	90	. Normal sinus rhythm, rate 90
PR	159	. Consider anterior infarct
QRSD	85	. Anterolateral ST-T abnormalities
QT	327	. Possible ischemia
QTc	400	. Probable inferior subepicardial injury

--AXIS--
P	58
QRS	66
T	92

- ABNORMAL ECG -

Normal P axis, PR, rate and rhythm   DOB:
Diminished R in V3 < 0.15 mV
ST > negative in I, aVL, V2-V6   MR:
T > -.30 mV, ST > -.05 mv
ST > .20 mV II, III, aVF

PRELIMINARY-MD MUST REVIEW

168

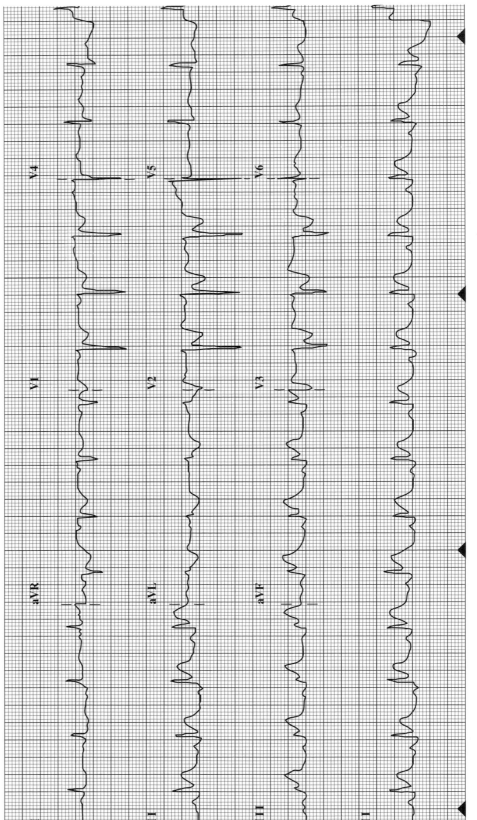

Figure 9–3. Subsequent 12-lead ECG performed 30 minutes after administration of streptokinase. Note the improvement in ST segment abnormalities from the previous study.

Mechanisms of Action (Why)

Plasmin is a fibrinolytic enzyme which, when formed close to a thrombus, will digest the fibrin strands that organize it. In this way the clot is dissolved.

Thrombolytic agents cleave soluble plasminogen into plasmin. The result is thrombolysis. There are four currently approved agents available:

- Streptokinase
- Urokinase
- Anistreplase
- Alteplase (TPA)

All of these four agents, are felt to be *equally effective* in reducing mortality.

Alteplase, also known as *tissue plasminogen activator (TPA), is a genetically engineered thrombolytic that activates surface-bound plasminogen. Because this plasmin is specific for clot fibrin, bleeding-related side effects should be measurably less.*

Indications (When)

Thrombolytic agents are indicated when there is ECG evidence that the patient is myocardially infarcting. This evidence is an ST segment elevation of 1 mm or greater in two contiguous leads on a 12-lead ECG in the setting of AMI.

- **Class I indications.** Patients meeting ECG criteria who are less than 70 years of age with signs and symptoms of less than 6 hours' duration and no absolute or relative contraindications.
- **Class IIa and IIb indications.** Patients older than 70 years with signs and symptoms of 6 to 12 hours' duration with no absolute and few relative contraindications.

Dosage (How)

Because the hazard of bleeding is so pronounced, thrombolytic agents are usually administered via a separate IV line.

- **Alteplase (TPA).** Give 60 mg IV in first hour (of which 6 to 10 mg is given initially IV push), and then 20 mg/hr for 2 additional hours.
- **Anistreplase.** 30 units IV over 2 to 5 min.
- **Streptokinase.** 1.5 million units in a 1-hr infusion.
- **Urokinase.** 1.5 million units over 2 min; followed by 1.5 million units over 90 min.

Absolute and Relative Contraindications

Bleeding is the hazard associated with thrombolytic agents. The list of absolute and relative contraindications below reflects this fact.

- *Absolute* contraindications for thrombolytic therapy:
    Active internal bleeding
    Suspected aortic dissection
    Known traumatic CPR
    Severe persistent hypertension despite pain relief and initial drugs
      (greater than 180 systolic or 110 diastolic)
    Recent head trauma or known intracranial neoplasm
    History of cerebrovascular accident in the past 6 months
    Pregnancy
- *Relative* contraindications:
    Recent trauma or major surgery in the past 2 months
    Initial blood pressure greater than 180 systolic or 110 diastolic
      that is controlled by medical treatment
    Active peptic ulcer or guaiac-positive stools
    History of cerebrovascular accident, tumor, injury, or brain surgery
    Known bleeding disorder or current use of warfarin
    Significant liver dysfunction or renal failure
    Exposure to streptokinase or anistreplase during the preceding 12
      months (these agents only)
    Known cancer or illness with possible thoracic, abdominal, or in-
      tracranial abnormalities
    Prolonged CPR

Heparin (IV)

Mechanisms of Action (Why)

Heparin, along with aspirin and thrombolytic agents, is considered part of the so-called *thrombolytic triad*. Even after effective lysis has occurred, the conditions that led to thrombus formation may still exist. Vascular injury and ruptured plaque surfaces can generate a fresh thrombus.

The value of heparin in the setting of AMI is that it prevents recurrence of thrombi *after* the performance of thrombolysis.

Indications (When)

- Heparin IV is *mandatory* with alteplase (TPA).
- Heparin is not necessary with anistreplase.
- Subcutaneous heparin is probably the optimal route with streptokinase.

Dosage for AMI (How)

A bolus of 5,000 units is given, followed by 1,000 units/hr for 24 to 48 hours. The dose should be adjusted to maintain an activated partial thromboplastin time (PTT) 1.5 to 2.0 times control values.

Hazards

In general, these are the same as those that apply to the use of thrombolytics.

- Active bleeding
- Recent surgery
- Presence of bleeding disorders

Beta Blockers

Mechanisms of Action (Why)

Research has shown that beta blockers given within the first 4 to 6 hours post-AMI and continued for 1 to 2 years can reduce mortality by about 33%. The therapeutic actions of the beta blockers are felt to reduce infarct size. They include:

- Decreased sinus node automaticity
- Lower blood pressure
- Decrease in myocardial oxygen demands

Indications for AMI (When)

In the context of AMI, beta blockers are useful in reducing the size of infarct. This is particularly true in patients with tachyarrhythmias and systemic hypertension.

Dosage for AMI (How)

- **Metoprolol.** 5 mg slow IV at 5-min intervals to a total of 15 mg.
- **Atenolol.** 5 mg slow IV (over 5 min). Wait 10 min, then give second dose of 5 mg slow IV (over 5 min).
- **Propanolol.** 1 mg slow IV every 5 min to a total of 5 mg.

Hazards

Because of the many potential side effects listed below, these agents must be administered with great caution in the setting of AMI.

- Bradycardia
- First- and second-degree type I AV block
- Hypotension
- Bronchospasm
- Worsening of CHF

Lidocaine

Mechanisms of Action (Why)

Lidocaine is a *first-line* agent for suppression of ventricular ectopy. It raises the fibrillatory threshold by decreasing the rate of automaticity of ectopic pacemakers and slowing conduction through re-entrant pathways.

Indications for AMI (When)

- Lidocaine is *not* indicated in the *routine prophylaxis* of PVCs.
- Lidocaine is *not* indicated to treat infrequent or asymptomatic PVCs. In the setting of AMI these are best managed with oxygen, nitroglycerin, morphine, or other modalities aimed at underlying ischemia.

Dosage for AMI (How)

- **Initial dose:** 1.0 to 1.5 mg/kg IV push. Additional boluses of 0.5–1.5 mg/kg can be given each 5 to 10 min.
- **Maximum dose:** 3 mg/kg.
- **Continuous infusion dose:** 2 to 4 mg/min.

Hazards

- Prophylactic use in AMI is *not* advised.
- Use with caution in patients with impaired liver function and reduced left ventricular function.

Magnesium Sulfate (IV)

Mechanisms of Action (Why)

Magnesium has the following actions that are felt to be beneficial to the patient with AMI:

- Antiarrhythmic actions
- Improves "electrical stability" of myocardium

Indications for AMI (When)

Magnesium sulfate is a class I (definitely helpful) agent in AMI occurring in patients with known or *suspected* magnesium deficiency.

This state is related strongly to poor nutritional status. It should be suspected in:

- Skilled nursing facility (SNF) admits
- Intravenous drug abusers and alcoholics
- Patients with chronic major organ insufficiency

Dosage for AMI (How)

Loading dose of 1 to 2 g over 5 to 60 min. Follow with 0.5 to 1.0 g/hr for up to 24 hr.

Hazards

- Use with caution in patients who are in renal failure.
- Rapid administration is associated with hypotension.

Percutaneous Transluminal Coronary Angioplasty (PTCA)

Mechanisms of Action (Why)

Balloon angioplasty can provide mechanical reperfusion of occluded arteries. Used in conjunction with sleevelike "stent" devices, this procedure is associated with a very low rate of reocclusion of the infarct-related artery. This procedure is performed in centers with a catheterization laboratory and a specially trained team.

Indications (When)

- Patients in whom thrombolytic therapy is contraindicated who have experienced a possible AMI for less than 6 hours (class I).
- Patients with AMI who develop cardiogenic shock within 18 hours after onset of symptoms (class IIa).
- Patients with a previous coronary artery bypass graft and suspected fresh occlusion.

AGENTS OF THE ACUTE PULMONARY EDEMA/HYPOTENSION/SHOCK ALGORITHM

Overview

The acute pulmonary edema/hypotension/shock algorithm (Figure 9–4) focuses on two of the most severe complications of AMI. *Cardiogenic shock* and *acute pulmonary edema* are most effectively treated when management can be guided by measurements available from catheterization of the

Acute Pulmonary Edema/Hypotension/Shock Algorithm

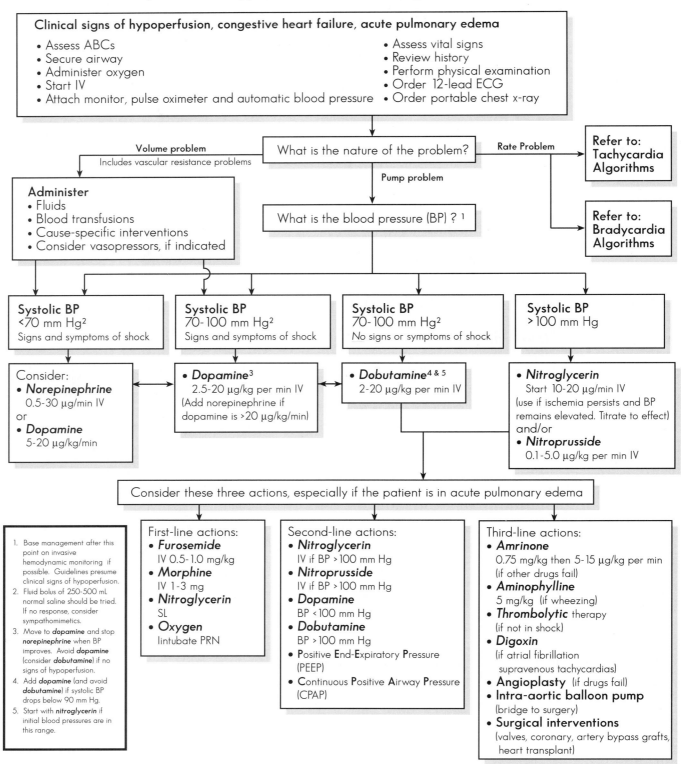

Figure 9–4. The acute pulmonary edema/hypotension/shock algorithm. This critical pathway details the management of AMI complicated by cardiogenic shock and acute pulmonary edema. This critical pathway is assessed in Case 10, Hypotension/Shock/Pulmonary Edema. (Algorithm copyright 1992, American Medical Association; JAMA, October 28, 1992; pp 2199–2241.)

pulmonary artery. It is generally accepted that when the *pulmonary wedge pressure* exceeds 18 mm Hg, clinical signs and symptoms of pulmonary congestion become apparent.

Similarly, when the *cardiac index* falls below 2.2 L/min/m², bedside evidence of peripheral hypoperfusion manifest themselves.

During ACLS, these hemodynamic measurements are not routinely available. Thus, these twin "pump problems" must be managed through evaluation of clinical markers of congestive heart failure. These classic findings are listed below.

Signs and Symptoms of Acute Pulmonary Edema (APE)

- Respiratory distress is the *cardinal sign* of APE
- Basal then global rales
- Third heart sound
- Radiologic evidence of pulmonary congestion
- Jugular venous distention (JVD)
- Pink frothy sputum

Signs and Symptoms of Cardiogenic Shock (Low Cardiac Output)

- Signs
  Chest pain
  Depressed mental status
- Symptoms
  Hypotension
  Weak pulse
  Cold diaphoretic skin
  Mottling and cyanosis of extremities
  Decreased urine output

Norepinephrine

Mechanisms of Action (Why)

Norepinephrine is a naturally occurring sympathomimetic agent that is used to increase blood pressure and maintain cardiac output. It possesses a powerful vasopressor (alpha-1) action. It also possesses a strong inotropic (beta-1) action.

Indications (When)

Norepinephrine is the agent for patients in cardiogenic shock who are unable to maintain a systolic BP greater than 70 mm Hg despite dopamine. It is *not* indicated to treat hypotension that is the result of hypovolemia.

Thus, the algorithm recommends a fluid bolus be given prior to administration of this drug.

Dosage (How)

The dosage of norepinephrine is 0.5 to 30 µg/min titrated to achieve a systolic BP in the range of 90 mm Hg.

Hazards

- **Arrhythmias.** At higher doses, norepinephrine's chronotropic side effects increase myocardial oxygen demand.
- **Arterial hypertension.** Increased systemic vascular resistance may have a deleterious effect on cardiac output and infarct size.

Dopamine

Mechanisms of Action (Why)

Dopamine is a sympathomimetic agent used to improve both blood pressure and cardiac output. Dopamine is a biochemical precursor of norepinephrine. It stimulates *dopaminergic*, beta-1, and alpha-1 receptors in a *dose-dependent* fashion that is outlined below.

- **Actions at "renal" doses.** In low doses (1 to 5 µg/kg/min) dilatation of renal and mesenteric arteries is caused by stimulation of *dopaminergic receptors.* Beta-1 and alpha-1 receptors are generally *not* affected by "renal dopamine."
- **Actions at "cardiac" doses.** In the dosage range of 5 to 10 µg/kg/min, dopamine produces *considerable* stimulation of beta-1 receptors with only *modest* alpha-1 activity. The result is usually an enhancement of cardiac output with only minimal increases in systemic vascular resistance.
- **Actions at "vasopressor" doses.** At doses above 10 µg/kg/min, the alpha-1 (vasopressor) actions of dopamine predominate. This usually results in *moderate* to *marked* increases in systemic vascular resistance.

Indications (When)

- Dopamine is the agent of choice for patients *with* signs and symptoms of cardiogenic shock whose systolic BP is in the range of 70 to 100 mm Hg. Hypotension due to hypovolemia should be ruled out with a volume infusion prior to dopamine administration.

- IV agent of second choice (after atropine) for hemodynamically unstable bradycardias.

Dosage (How)

- **Renal (low) doses.** 1 to 5 μg/kg/min
- **Cardiac (moderate) doses.** 5 to 10 μg/kg/min
- **Vasopressor (high) doses.** 10 to 20 μg/kg/min

Hazards

- **Arrhythmias.** At higher doses chronotropic side effects can induce arrhythmias by increasing myocardial oxygen demands.
- **Hypertension.** Overadministration can lead to pronounced increases in systemic vascular resistance. This can adversely affect infarct size and cardiac output.

Dobutamine

Mechanisms of Action (Why)

Dobutamine is a synthetic sympathomimetic agent. It exerts its potent inotropic actions by stimulating beta-1 receptors. It also produces mild stimulation of beta-2 receptors in vascular smooth muscle so that decreases in systemic vascular resistance are usually noted. Blood pressure usually is unchanged or even minimally increased due to improvements in cardiac output.

Indications (When)

Dobutamine is the agent of choice for patients *without* signs and symptoms of cardiogenic shock whose blood pressure is in the range of 70 to 100 mm Hg. Hypotension due to hypovolemia should be ruled out with a volume infusion prior to administering dobutamine.

When the BP is between 70 and 90 mm Hg, dopamine should be added as a safety precaution.

Dosage (How)

Dobutamine is given 2 to 20 μg/kg/min. Titrate to achieve a systolic blood pressure in the range of 90 mm Hg so that the heart rate does not increase greater than 10% from baseline.

Hazards

- **Arrhythmias.** At higher doses, dobutamine's chronotropic actions are often pronounced. This can substantially increase myocardial oxygen demand and worsen ischemia.

Nitroglycerin and Nitroprusside

Mechanisms of Action (Why)

These nitrate-based agents are valuable in the treatment of cardiogenic shock because of their beneficial hemodynamic effects. They both dilate arteriolar smooth muscle. This makes them valuable in lowering the left ventricular workloads in patients with systolic BP greater than 100 mm Hg. To a lesser extent, these drugs also dilate venular smooth muscle. This decreases venous return to the right heart and helps reduce pulmonary congestion.

In the setting of AMI complicated by pump failure, IV nitroglycerin is generally preferred over nitroprusside.

Indications (When)

- Both drugs are indicated to treat pump failure complicated by systolic blood pressures greater then 100 mm Hg.
- Both drugs effectively reduce left heart afterload in the setting of complicated acute MI.
- Nitroglycerin is usually preferred during the first 30 to 60 minutes post-AMI.
- Nitroprusside is often chosen during the *post-resuscitation phase* where hemodynamic monitoring renders unwanted swings in blood pressure less likely.

Dosage (How)

- **Nitroglycerin.** 10 to 20 μg/min, titrated to effect.
- **Nitroprusside.** Begin at 0.1 μg/kg per min and titrate upward every 3 to 5 min to desired effect (up to 5 μg/kg per min).

Hazards

- **Hypotension.** The major complication of both nitroglycerin and nitroprusside is hypotension. With both drugs, systolic blood pressures less than 90 mm Hg should be avoided.

Furosemide

Mechanisms of Action (Why)

Furosemide is one of the stalwarts in the treatment of acute pulmonary edema. It possesses two actions which make it a first-line agent. *First,* it dilates venous smooth muscle, causing venous return to the right heart to decrease. This action occurs within five minutes of administration.

Second, furosemide also produces a strong diuresis by inhibiting reabsorbtion of sodium in the loop of Henle and in the tubules. Diuresis begins within minutes and reaches a peak in 30 minutes.

Indications (When)

First-line agent for AMI complicated by acute pulmonary edema. See Figure 9–4.

Dosage (How)

Furosemide is given 0.5 to 1.0 mg/kg slow IV push; if no response, give 2 mg/kg slow IV push.

Hazards

- **Hypotension.** Furosemide should generally not be administered if the systolic BP is less than 90 mm Hg.
- **Dehydration**
- **Electrolyte disturbances**

AGENTS OF THE VF/VT AND TACHYCARDIA ALGORITHMS (FOR SUPPRESSION OF VENTRICULAR ECTOPY)

Overview

Figures 9–5 and 9–6, the VF/VT and stable tachycardia algorithms, recommend the following four IV medications for their value in suppressing ventricular ectopy. These agents may be used to treat PVCs, ventricular tachycardia, and ventricular fibrillation.

- Lidocaine
- Procainamide
- Bretylium
- Magnesium sulfate

Ventricular Fibrillation/Pulseless Ventricular Tachycardia (VF/VT) Algorithm

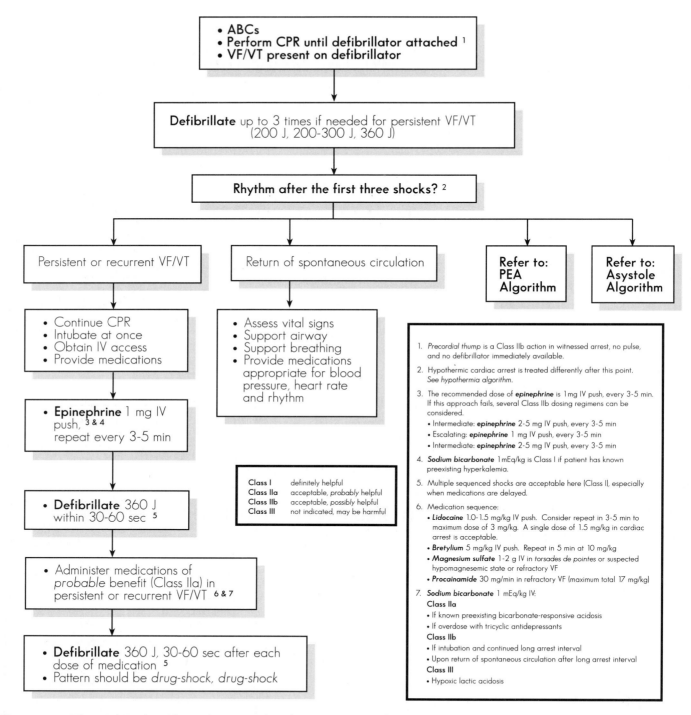

Figure 9–5. The VF/VT algorithm. This critical pathway is assessed in Case 3, Mega VF: Refractory VF/Pulseless VT. (Algorithm copyright 1992, American Medical Association; JAMA, October 28, 1992; pp 2199–2241.)

Tachycardia Algorithm

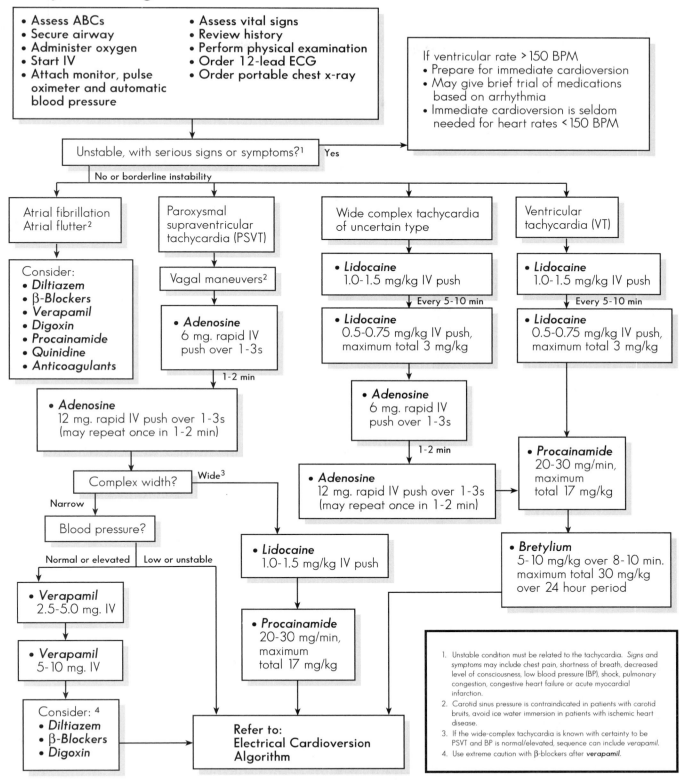

Figure 9–6. The stable tachycardia algorithm. This critical pathway is assessed in Case 9, Stable Tachycardia. (Algorithm copyright 1992, American Medical Association; JAMA, October 28, 1992; pp 2199–2241.)

Lidocaine

Mechanisms of Action (Why)

Lidocaine is a *first-line* agent in the suppression of ventricular ectopy. Lidocaine raises the fibrillatory threshold by:

- Decreasing the rate of automaticity of ectopic pacemaker cells.
- Slowing conduction through re-entrant pathways.

Indications (When)

- Cardiac arrest due to VF and/or pulseless VT that is refractory to defibrillation and epinephrine (see VF/VT algorithm).
- *Stable* VT (systolic BP > 80 mm Hg).
- *Stable* wide-complex tachycardias of uncertain type (systolic BP > 80 mm Hg).
- Symptomatic PVCs (frequent, multiformed, salvos, etc. that do not respond to oxygen, morphine, and nitroglycerin).

Dosage (How)

- **Cardiac arrest from VF/VT.** Initial dose 1.0 to 1.5 mg/kg IV push. For refractory VF/VT, may repeat at 1.0 to 1.5 mg/kg in 3 to 5 min; maximum total 3 mg/kg.
- **Ventricular ectopy.** 1.0 to 1.5 mg/kg IV push. Repeat at 0.5 to 0.75 mg/kg every 5 to 10 min; maximum total 3 mg/kg.
- **Maintenance infusion.** 2 to 4 mg/min (30 to 50 µg/kg per min).

Hazards

- Prophylactic use in AMI is *not* recommended.
- Use with caution in patients with impaired liver function and reduced left ventricular function.

Procainamide

Mechanisms of Action (Why)

Procainamide is a *second-line* antiarrhythmic agent (after lidocaine). Procainamide raises the fibrillatory threshold by:

- Reducing the rate of automaticity of ectopic pacemakers.
- Slowing intraventricular conduction and terminating re-entrant arrhythmias.

Indications (When)

- Refractory VF/VT not responsive to:
  Defibrillation
  Epinephrine
  Lidocaine
  Bretylium
- Stable VT not responsive to lidocaine
- Stable wide-complex tachycardia of unknown origin not responsive to lidocaine or adenosine.

Dosage (How)

- **VF/VT.** 30 mg/min (maximum total, 17 mg/kg)
- **Stable tachycardias.** 20 to 30 mg/min until one of following is noted:
  Arrhythmia suppression
  Hypotension
  QRS widens greater than 50%
  Total of 17 mg/kg given
- **Maintenance infusion.** 1 to 4 mg/min

Hazards

- Procainamide is contraindicated when pre-existing QT prolongation and/or *Torsade de pointes* are present.
- Hypotension

Bretylium

Mechanisms of Action (Why)

Bretylium is a complex pharmacologic agent that is useful in the treatment of refractory VF/VT. It possesses several beneficial mechanisms that act in concert to produce its beneficial actions. Listed below, they include:

- An initial release of catecholamines upon injection.
- A beta-blocking action that develops 5 to 10 minutes post administration.
- A possible antiarrhythmic action.

Indications (When)

- Refractory VF/VT not responsive to:
  Defibrillation
  Epinephrine
  Lidocaine
- Stable VT not responding to lidocaine or procainamide.

Dosage (How)

- **Refractory VF/VT.** 5 mg/kg IV bolus. Repeat at 10 mg/kg in 5 min. Maximum dose 30 to 35 mg/kg.
- **Stable VT.** 5 to 10 mg/kg over 8 to 10 min. Wait 10 to 30 min before next dose. Maximum 30 mg/kg over 24 hours.

Hazards

- Hypotension

Magnesium Sulfate

Mechanisms of Action (Why)

Magnesium deficiency can trigger recurrent ventricular arrhythmias, including *Torsade de pointes* and VF. Magnesium as a drug has antiarrhythmic properties that are believed to be related to its ability to provide for and preserve electrical stability in the myocardium.

Indications (When)

- Cardiac arrest associated with Torsade de pointes or suspected magnesium deficiency.
- Refractory VF (after lidocaine, bretylium, and procainamide).
- Nonpulseless Torsade de pointes.

Dosage (How)

- **Refractory VF/VT.** Loading dose of 1 to 2 g IV over 1 to 2 min.
- **Torsade de pointes.** Loading dose of 1 to 2 g IV over 1 to 2 min.
- **Acute myocardial infarction.** Loading dose of 1 to 2 gm IV administered over 5–60 minutes.

Hazards

- Hypotension

AGENTS OF THE TACHYCARDIA ALGORITHM (FOR SUPPRESSION OF ATRIAL ECTOPY)

Overview

The stable tachycardia algorithm (Figure 9–6) presents recommendations for pharmacologic management of paroxysmal supraventricular tachycardia

(PSVT), atrial flutter, atrial fibrillation, and wide-complex tachycardias of uncertain type. Recommended agents to be covered in an essential ACLS provider course are as follows:

- Vagal maneuvers
- Adenosine
- Diltiazem and verapamil
- Beta blockers

Vagal Maneuvers

Mechanisms of Action (Why)

PSVT relies on a re-entrant pathway that cycles impulses rapidly through the AV node. Stimulation of vagal fibers results in slowing of conduction through the AV node. This frequently results in conversion of PSVT to a sinus rhythm.

Of the many techniques for stimulation described, *carotid sinus massage* and *facial ice water immersion* are most commonly employed. Not without their hazards, these techniques should be used only when ECG monitoring and IV access are available.

Indications (When)

Vagal maneuvers are indicated in the treatment of PSVT. They are *not* recommended for *treatment* of atrial fibrillation or atrial flutter. In atrial flutter, carotid sinus pressure may make F waves more electrocardiographically visible. The diagnosis may be confirmed in this way.

Hazards

- Cartoid sinus pressure is contraindicated in patients with *cartoid bruits* or other substantial evidence of cerebral vascular disease.
- Facial ice water immersion should be avoided in patients with ischemic heart disease.
- Valsalva-type maneuvers may be employed when other vagal maneuvers are less advisable.

Adenosine

Mechanisms of Action (Why)

Adenosine acts directly to slow conduction through the fibers of the AV node. Since PSVT usually owes its existence to a re-entry circuit involving the AV node, this arrhythmia is often terminated by administration.

Indications (When)

As reflected in the tachycardia algorithm, the JAMA guidelines recommend adenosine as the *agent of first choice* for stable PSVT. Also favoring the first-line status of this agent is the fact that it produces hypotension less frequently than verapamil (the agent of second choice for PSVT).

In addition, because of its very short (5 to 10 sec) half-life, side effects tend to be transient.

A close look at the tachycardia algorithm reveals that adenosine is the *second-line agent* for stable wide-complex tachycardias of uncertain type. Here this drug is of value in distinguishing supraventricular from ventricular tachycardia.

Dosage (How)

- 6 mg, rapid IV push (over 1 to 3 sec).
- If no response in 1 to 2 min; 12 mg rapid IV push (over 1 to 3 sec).
- This dosage may be repeated in 1 to 2 min if conversion has not occurred.

Hazards

Hazards are usually transient owing to the brief half-life of the agent. They include:

- Hypotension (patients are usually placed in a mild reverse Trendelenburg)
- Bradyarrhythmias
- Ventricular ectopy
- Transient chest pain, flushing, and shortness of breath

Verapamil

Mechanisms of Action (Why)

Verapamil is a calcium channel-blocking agent. It inhibits calcium ions from flowing into myocardial and vascular smooth muscle cells. This results in the following actions.

- **Decrease in systemic vascular resistance.** Unwanted hypotension can be a problem.
- **Potent negative *chronotropic* effect.** The rate of sinus node automaticity is decreased.
- **Pronounced negative *dromotropic* effect.** Verapamil slows conduction through the AV node.
- **Potent negative *inotropic* effect.** It will depress myocardial function of patients with pump failure.

Indications (When)

- Verapamil is the *second-line agent* (after adenosine for treatment of narrow complex PSVT).
- Verapamil is a *third-line agent* for controlling the ventricular rate in atrial flutter and atrial fibrillation. Its more pronounced depressive effect on vascular and myocardial muscle tone make it a less desirable agent than diltiazem or beta blockers.

Dosage (How)

Verapamil is given as a 2.5 to 5.0 mg IV bolus over 1 to 2 min. Repeat 5 to 10 mg, if needed, in 15 to 30 min; maximum dose 30 mg.

Hazards

- Verapamil, and other calcuim channel-blocking agents, are class III (*probably harmful*) agents in the treatment of both VT *and* wide-complex tachycardias of uncertain origin.
- The risk of hypotension is more pronounced with verapamil than with diltiazem.
- Do not use with *oral* or *IV* beta blockers.

Diltiazem

Mechanisms of Action (Why)

Diltiazem, like verapamil, is a calcium channel-blocking agent. It inhibits calcium ions from flowing into myocardial and vascular smooth muscle cells. This results in the following:

- Decreases in systemic vascular resistance that are *less pronounced* than with verapamil.
- Potent negative *chronotropic* effects that are *similar* to verapamil.
- Pronounced negative *dromotropic* effects *similar* to verapamil.
- Negative *inotropic* effects that are *less pronounced* than seen with verapamil.

Indications (When)

- *First-line* agent to slow ventricular rate in atrial flutter and atrial fibrillation.

Dosage (How)

Diltiazem is given 15 to 20 mg (0.25 mg/kg) IV over 2 min. May repeat in 15 min at 20 to 25 mg (0.35 mg/kg) over 2 min.

Hazards

- Diltiazem and other calcium channel-blocking agents are class III (*probably harmful*) agents for the management of VT and wide-complex tachycardias of uncertain origin.
- Hypotension is less common with diltiazem than with verapamil but is still a fairly common side effect.
- Do not use with *oral* or *IV* beta blockers.

Beta Blockers (Metoprolol, Propranolol, Atenolol, Esmolol)

Mechanisms of Action (Why)

This group of agents have useful actions in the setting of ACLS because of their ability to blunt stimulation of the heart's beta-1 adrenergic receptors.

Propranolol, the prototype, provides nonselective blockade of both beta-1 and beta-2 receptors. Thus, in addition to providing negative chronotropic, negative dromotropic, and negative inotropic cardiac actions, it must also be used with caution in patients with asthma, and in patients with a systolic BP less than 100 mm Hg.

Atenolol, metoprolol, and esmolol selectively block only beta-1 receptor sites. With these agents, beta-2-related side effects are not seen until higher doses are used.

Indications (When)

- Atrial flutter and atrial fibrillation not responding to other therapies. *Note*: These agents should *not* be administered concurrently with calcium channel blockers, as side effects are similar.
- Research has shown that beta blockers given within the first 4 to 6 hours post-AMI and continued for 1 to 2 years can reduce mortality by as much as 33%.

Dosage (How)

- **Esmolol.** Loading dose of 250 to 500 μg/kg for 1 min, followed by a maintenance dose of 25 to 50 μg/kg/min given for 4 min. The final infusion rate is titrated to effect to a maximum dose of 300 μg/kg/min.
- **Metoprolol.** 5 mg slow IV at 5-min intervals to a total of 15 mg.
- **Atenolol.** 5 mg slow IV (over 5 min). Wait 10 min, then give second dose of 5 mg slow IV (over 5 min). In 10 min, if tolerated well, may start 50 mg PO, then give 50 mg PO BID.
- **Propranolol.** 1 to 3 mg slow IV. Do not exceed 1 mg/min. Repeat a second dose after 2 min, if necessary.

Hazards

In the contex of ACLS the following hazards must be guarded against.
- Bradycardia
- First- and second-degree type I AV block
- Hypotension
- Bronchospasm
- Worsening of CHF

AGENTS RECOMMENDED IN THE BRADYCARDIA ALGORITHM

Overview

The bradycardia algorithm (Figure 9–7) recommends that patients with either absolute or relative bradycardias who are *symptomatic* be managed using the following intervention sequence:

- Atropine 0.5 to 1.0 mg IV push (classes I and IIa)
- Transcutaneous pacemaker (class I)
- Dopamine infusion at 5 to 20 µg/kg/min (class IIb)
- Epinephrine infusion at 2 to 10 µg/min (class IIb)
- Isoproterenol infusion (classes IIb and III)

Atropine

Mechanisms of Action (Why)

The action of this agent is to block impulses from the parasympathetic branch of the autonomic nervous system. This results in the following actions which make it useful in treating symptomatic bradycardias:

- **Positive *chronotropic* effect.** The rate of automaticity of pacemaker cells in the sinus node is accelerated; thus, a bradycardic rhythm may be abolished.
- **Positive *dromotropic* effect.** Conduction of impulses through the AV node is enhanced. As a result, arrhythmias such as first- and second-degree type I AV blocks are frequently amenable to this drug.

Indications (When)

- Atropine is the *first-line IV agent* for symptomatic bradycardias.
- As a *temporizing agent* until a pacemaker can be placed. Second-degree type II and third-degree AV blocks typically require a transvenous pacemaker. Temporizing, first with atropine and then with a transcutaneous pacemaker (TCP), is required while preparations are made to perform this invasive procedure.

Bradycardia Algorithm
(Patient is not in cardiac arrest)

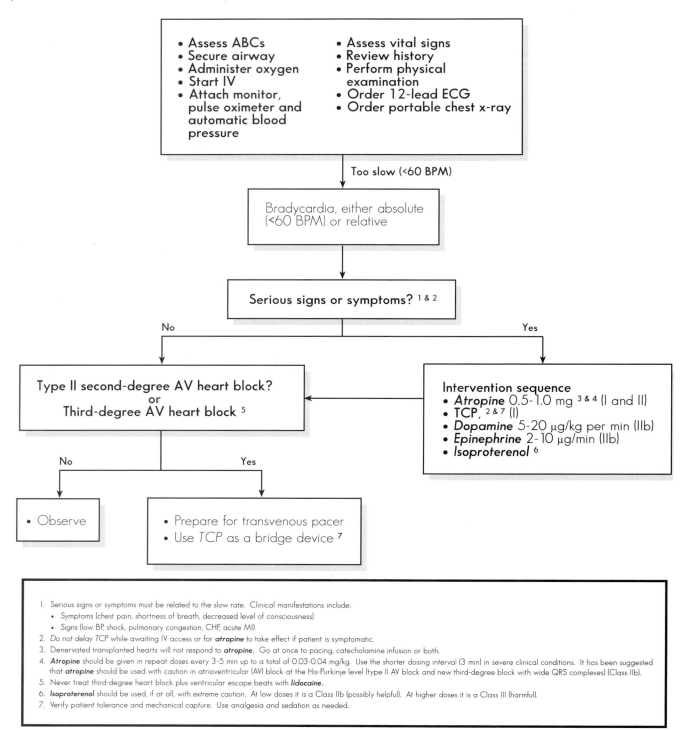

- Assess ABCs
- Secure airway
- Administer oxygen
- Start IV
- Attach monitor, pulse oximeter and automatic blood pressure
- Assess vital signs
- Review history
- Perform physical examination
- Order 12-lead ECG
- Order portable chest x-ray

Too slow (<60 BPM)

Bradycardia, either absolute (<60 BPM) or relative

Serious signs or symptoms? [1 & 2]

No

Type II second-degree AV heart block?
or
Third-degree AV heart block [5]

No

- Observe

Yes

- Prepare for transvenous pacer
- Use *TCP* as a bridge device [7]

Yes

Intervention sequence
- *Atropine* 0.5-1.0 mg [3 & 4] (I and II)
- TCP, [2 & 7] (I)
- *Dopamine* 5-20 µg/kg per min (IIb)
- *Epinephrine* 2-10 µg/min (IIb)
- *Isoproterenol* [6]

1. Serious signs or symptoms must be related to the slow rate. Clinical manifestations include:
   - *Symptoms* (chest pain, shortness of breath, decreased level of consciousness)
   - *Signs* (low BP, shock, pulmonary congestion, CHF, acute MI)
2. *Do not delay TCP* while awaiting IV access or for *atropine* to take effect if patient is symptomatic.
3. Denervated transplanted hearts will not respond to *atropine*. Go at once to pacing, catecholamine infusion or both.
4. *Atropine* should be given in repeat doses every 3-5 min up to a total of 0.03-0.04 mg/kg. Use the shorter dosing interval (3 min) in severe clinical conditions. It has been suggested that *atropine* should be used with caution in atrioventricular (AV) block at the His-Purkinje level (type II AV block and new third-degree block with wide QRS complexes) (Class IIb).
5. Never treat third-degree heart block plus ventricular escape beats with *lidocaine.*
6. *Isoproterenol* should be used, if at all, with *extreme caution.* At low doses it is a Class IIb (possibly helpful). At higher doses it is a Class III (harmful).
7. Verify patient tolerance and mechanical *capture.* Use analgesia and sedation as needed.

Figure 9–7. The bradycardia algorithm. This critical pathway is evaluated in Case 7, Bradycardia. (Algorithm copyright 1992, American Medical Association; JAMA, October 28, 1992; pp 2199–2241.)

- Cardiac arrest due to asystole or bradycardic PEA (class IIb). Atropine is the second-line IV agent. It is used *after* epinephrine.

Dosage (How)

- **Asystole or slow PEA.** 1 mg IV push. Repeat every 3 to 5 min (if asystole persists) to maximum dose of 0.04 mg/kg.
- **Symptomatic bradycardia.** 0.5 to 1.0 mg IV every 3 to 5 min as needed; not to exceed total dose of 0.04 mg/kg.
- **Endotracheal dose.** 1 to 2.5 mg diluted in 10 mL NS or distilled water.

Hazards

Because of its positive chronotropic effect, atropine increases myocardial oxygen demand. Thus, it should be used with caution in patients with myocardial ischemia and injury. The guidelines state that atropine should be used with caution in the following settings:

- Bradycardias due to AMI
- Patients with second-degree type II and third-degree AV blocks with broad QRS complexes

Transcutaneous Pacing

The guidelines state that transcutaneous pacing is a *class I* intervention in *all* aymptomatic bradycardias. These devices are used as a bridging mechanism in the management of second-degree type II and third-degree AV blocks until a transvenous pacemaker can be placed.

Dopamine and Epinephrine

A *dopamine infusion* at a rate of 5 to 20 µg/kg/min is a class IIb intervention.

It should be started promptly in patients who do not respond to atropine or TCP.

An epinephrine infusion at 2 to 10 µg/min is also a class IIb intervention. It is recommended when bradycardia and hypotension exist despite dopamine administration.

Isoproterenol at 2–10 µg/min

Isoproterenol is a synthetic sympathomimetic agent with pure beta-adrenergic stimulating properties. It is a remarkably powerful inotrope that also produces vasodilatation. Unfortunately, its positive chronotropic actions are so pronounced that its use is virtually synonymous with tachyarrhythmia formation. Both the JAMA guidelines and the bradycardia algorithm state that this is an agent of *last resort* which, if used at all, be administered with extreme caution.

With these caveats in mind isoproterenol is a IIb intervention at lower doses. It is a class III (harmful) intervention at higher doses.

BIBLIOGRAPHY

1. American Heart Association. Emergency Cardiac Care Committee and Subcommittees. Guidelines for cardiopulmonary resuscitation and emergency cardiac care. JAMA 1992;268:2171–2295
2. American Heart Association. Textbook of advanced cardiac life support. Dallas, TX: American Heart Association, 1994
3. American Heart Association. Instructor's manual for advanced cardiac life support. Dallas, TX: American Heart Association, 1994
4. ACC/AHA Task Force Report. Guidelines for the early management of patients with acute myocardial infarction: a report of the American College of Cardiology/American Heart Association Task Force on Assessment of Diagnosis and Therapeutic Cardiovascular Procedures (subcommittee to develop guidelines for the early management of patients with acute myocardial infarction). J Am Coll Cardiol 1990;16:249–292
5. Eisenberg MS, Aghababian RV, Bossaert L, Jaffe AS, Ornato JP, Weaver WD. Thrombolytic therapy. Ann Emerg Med 1993;22(Part 2):417–427
6. Kette F, Weil MH, van Planta M, Gazmuri RJ, Rackow EC. Buffer agents do not reverse intramyocardial acidosis during cardiac resuscitation. Circulation 1990;81:1660–1666
7. Meischke H, Ho MT, Eisenberg MS, Schaeffer SM, Larsen MP. Reasons patients with chest pain delay or do not call 911. Ann Emerg Med, February 1995;25:193–197
8. Paraids NA, Martin GB, Rivers EP, Goetting MG, Appleton TJ, Feingold M, Nowak RM. Coronary perfusion pressure and the return of spontaneous circulation in human cardiopulmonary resuscitation. JAMA 1009;263:1106–1113
9. Rau JL. ACLS drugs used during resuscitation. Respir Care 1995;40:404–426

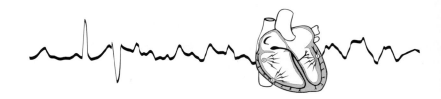

10. Lethal Arrhythmias

OUTLINE

Essential ACLS Curricula

Ventricular Fibrillation/Pulseless Ventricular
Tachycardia (VF/VT)

Asystole

Pulseless Electrical Activity (PEA)

Electrocardiographic Artifact

ESSENTIAL ACLS CURRICULA

Both ACLS and BLS guidelines make distinction between biologic and clinical death. The latter is said to exist whenever unresponsiveness, apnea, and pulselessness are present. These victims are also said to be in *cardiac arrest.*

Figure 10–1, the universal algorithm for adult ECG, directs that once pulselessness is determined and CPR is started, the patient's cardiac rhythm is to be evaluated on the monitor/defibrillator.

As depicted by the universal algorithm, there are three lethal "arrhythmias" responsible for cardiac arrest. As discussed in Chapters 2 and 3, ventricular fibrillation/pulseless ventricular tachycardia (VF/VT) is responsible for 80 to 90% of all episodes of cardiac arrest. This explains why the most important goal of ACLS is early defibrillation.

Asystole and pulseless electrical activity (PEA) are also responsible for cardiac arrest. PEA is defined as pulselessness and the presence of a rhythm *other* than VF/VT or asystole on the monitor. PEA is most often the result of treatable underlying causes such as *hypovolemia, hypoxia, cardiac tamponade,* and *tension pneumothorax.*

In contrast, asystole commonly represents the terminal efforts of a dy-

Universal Algorithm for Adult
Emergency Cardiac Care

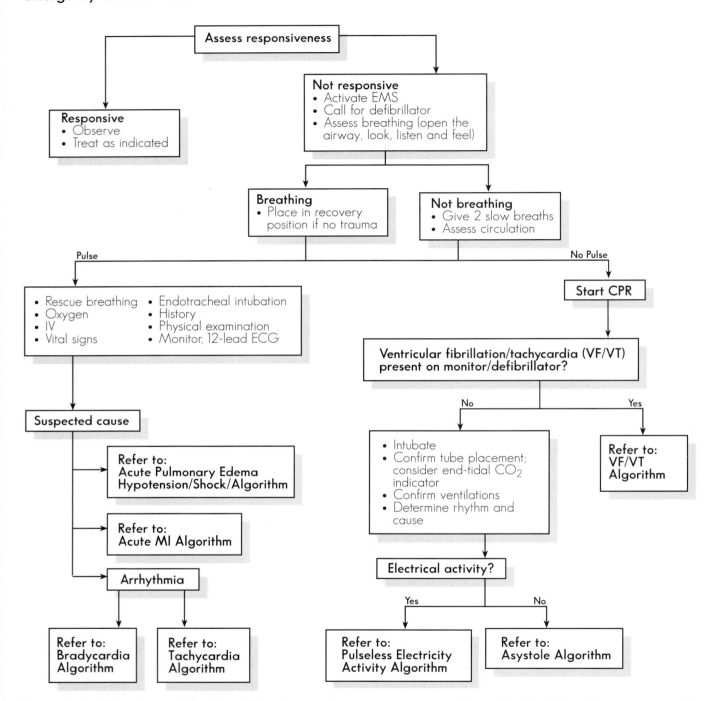

Figure 10–1. The universal algorithm. These intervention sequences are evaluated in Case I: Respiratory Arrest with a Pulse. (Algorithm copyright 1992, American Medical Association; JAMA, October 28, 1992; pp 2199–2241.)

ing heart. The guidelines state that asystole is often a confirmation of death rather than an actual rhythm to be treated.

No discussion of lethal arrhythmias would be complete without mentioning that both VF/VT and asystole can be mimicked by *electrocardiographic artifact*. The spectre of such a patient receiving electrical counter-shock is a potent reminder that the first and last rule of ACLS is "treat the patient, not the monitor."

VENTRICULAR FIBRILLATION/PULSELESS VENTRICULAR TACHYCARDIA (VF/VT)

Clinical Significance

Illustrated in Figure 10–2, VF/VT is responsible for the overwhelming majority of cases of cardiac arrest. Since defibrillation is the only definitive

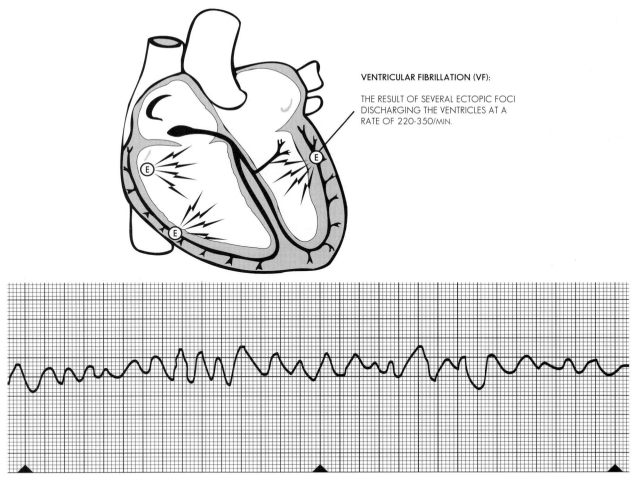

VENTRICULAR FIBRILLATION (VF):

THE RESULT OF SEVERAL ECTOPIC FOCI DISCHARGING THE VENTRICLES AT A RATE OF 220-350/MIN.

Figure 10–2. Ventricular fibrillation is responsible for 80 to 90% of episodes of cardiac arrest. The only definitive therapy for VF/pulseless VT is defibrillation.

therapy for this lethal rhythm, the cornerstone of ACLS is early defibrillation.

Description

The best word to describe VF is *chaotic*. There are no recognizable QRS complexes. P waves and T waves are not present. The only electrocardiographic manifestation is the presence of a highly irregular fibrillatory line. Clinicians describe these fibrillatory lines in terms of their amplitude. Higher amplitude, *coarse VF,* often signifies both recent onset and amenability to defibrillation. In contrast, *fine VF* tends to be both refractory to electrical countershock and generally signifies an arrest of considerable duration.

Figure 10–3 shows the progression of VF from coarse to fine over the span of several minutes.

Treatment

The therapeutic sequence outlined in the VF/VT algorithm (Figure 10–4) forms the core of adult ACLS. The steps deemed necessary to treat VF are as follows:

- **STEP 1:** Defibrillate times three if needed (200 to 300 J, 360 J)

  Immediately upon determining that VF/VT is present, defibrillation is to be performed. Because it is the definitive therapy, it is indicated even in instances where response time has been delayed.

  The guidelines are unequivocal. CPR must be stopped and no attempts made to deliver medications until three shocks have proved unsuccessful.

  These three unsynchronized shocks are to be delivered in a "stacked" manner with only enough time being taken in between to recharge the defibrillator and to confirm the presence or absence of VF/VT.

  During this time, the paddles are to be left pressed on the chest and personnel instructed to remain "clear." This means that pulse checks, CPR, etc., must *not* be performed at this time. Energy levels recommended for this sequence are:

    200 J
    200 to 300 J
    360 J

When performing defibrillation, efforts must be made to minimize *transthoracic impedance.* These include:

- Modern remote defibrillation systems
- Use of successive shocks
- Use of "paddle pressure"
- Use of conductive media between chest wall and electrodes

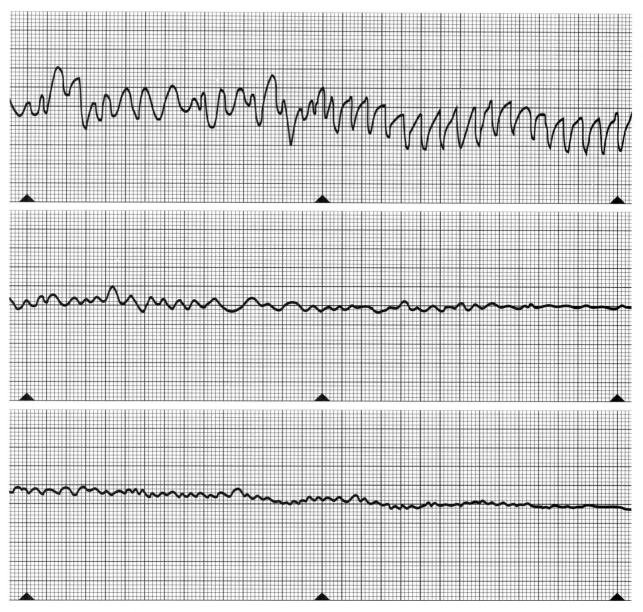

Figure 10–3. Progression of coarse VF into fine VF. Within minutes after onset, coarse electrical energy waveforms lose their amplitude and are reduced to a fine line that can be difficult to distinguish from asystole.

- **STEP 2:** Resume CPR, intubate immediately, and establish IV access. The patient who does not respond to these three initial attempts at defibrillation is said to have *refractory VF/VT.*

  Failure to respond to electrical countershock denotes the presence of considerable underlying pathology. The JAMA guidelines note that patient outcomes from this point on deteriorate markedly.

- **STEP 3:** Administer epinephrine 1.0 mg IV. Repeat as necessary each 3 to 5 min. Epinephrine increases myocardial and cerebral blood flow better than any other pharmacologic agent. This makes it the only class I (definitely helpful) drug for *all* pulseless rhythms.

Ventricular Fibrillation/Pulseless Ventricular Tachycardia (VF/VT) Algorithm

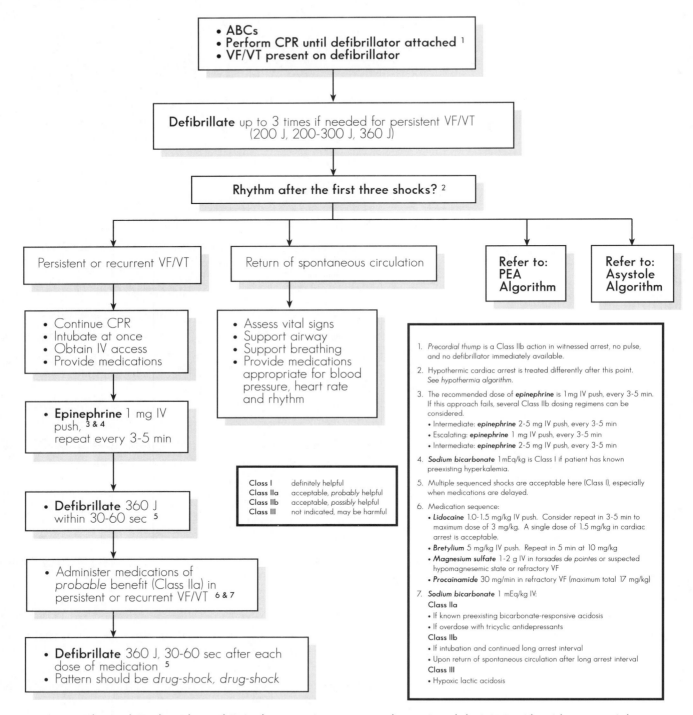

Figure 10–4. The VF/VT algorithm. This is the most important pathway in adult ACLS. (Algorithm copyright 1992, American Medical Association; JAMA, October 28, 1992; pp 2199–2241.)

During cardiac arrest, IV agents are usually administered via a vein in the antecubital fossa. The guidelines state that drug administration under these circumstances should be followed by a 20-mL fluid bolus and elevation of the extremity.

Epinephrine can be given endotracheally. The dose is 2.0 to 2.5 mg with 10 mL of NS.

- **STEP 4:** Defibrillate at 360 J within 30 to 60 sec if VF/VT is still present.

   Rescuers must allow 30 to 60 sec for IV drugs given during cardiac arrest to reach the central organs. During this time, the rhythm is reassessed. If VF/VT is still present, an unsynchronized countershock of 360 J is administered.

- **STEP 5:** Administer lidocaine 1.0 to 1.5 mg/kg IV push. This dose can be repeated in 3 to 5 min up to a maximum total of 3 mg/kg.

- **STEP 6:** Defibrillate at 360 J 30 to 60 sec after drug administration.

- **STEP 7:** Bretylium 5 mg/kg IV push. After 5 min, 10 mg/kg can be given. The maximum dose is 30 to 35 mg/kg.

- **STEP 8:** Defibrillate at 360 J 30 to 60 sec after drug administration.

- **STEP 9:** Procainamide 30 mg/min up to maximum dose of 17 mg/kg.

- **STEP 10:** Defibrillate at 360 J 30 to 60 sec after drug administration.

If VF/VT persists, continue to administer medications of probable benefit (IIa) followed by defibrillation at 360 J. The pattern should be: *drug–shock, drug–shock.*

Examples of VF/VT

Illustrated below are several examples of VF/VT. Figure 10–5 shows VF/VT being precipitated by an R wave which occurs during the relative refractory

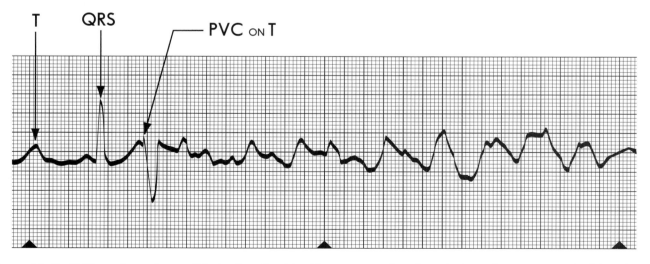

Figure 10–5. PVC on downslope of T. As described in Chapters 3 and 4, the relative refractory period of the electrographic cycle corresponds most closely to the downslope of the T wave. In this example, a PVC occurs during this vulnerable time and precipitates coarse VF.

R ON T

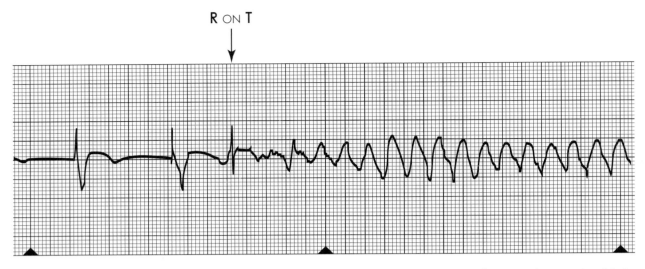

Figure 10–6. Onset of VF/VT. In this example, the first two complexes are junctional escape beats. The third complex is a premature junctional contraction (PJC), which is closely coupled to the previous T wave. The resulting rhythm is VF/VT.

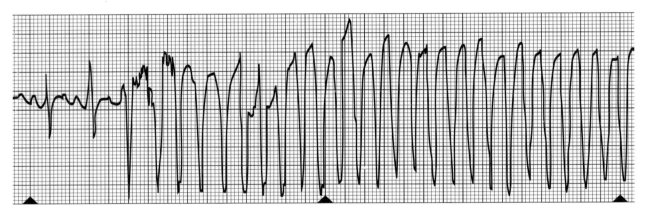

Figure 10–7. Onset of extremely rapid VF/VT. In this ECG, a PVC occurs after the T wave, triggering VT with a rate approaching 300/min. Delays in synchronization are very common in ventricular tachycardia when rates surpass 200/min. Pulselessness is common at high rates.

period of the electrophysiologic cycle. Similarly, Figure 10–6 depicts VF/VT being triggered by a PJC that is coupled closely to the previous T wave. Finally, Figure 10–7 illustrates the onset of a very rapid ventricular tachycardia. In this instance, the lethal rhythm was initiated by an R wave occurring just after the preceding T wave.

ASYSTOLE

Clinical Significance

The guidelines state that cardiac arrest due to ventricular asystole "most often represents a confirmation of death, rather than an actual rhythm to be treated."

If asystole persists despite appropriate therapy and if no underlying treatable causes can be found, the JAMA guidelines suggest that the team leader consider termination of code efforts (refer to Figure 10–8).

Description

Ventricular asystole is defined by the absence of ventricular complexes. Occasionally, atrial activity is present as can be seen in Figure 10–9.

Treatment

When confronted with a "flatline" on the monitor, the ACLS provider must rule out *false asystole* as a cause of the isoelectric line. This is most often due to operator error, although occasionally VF may present as an isoelectric line.

- Operator error:
  Loose leads
  No power
  Disconnected leads
- Isoelectric VF:
  Rarely VF may produce asystole in one lead. To rule out this possibility, the operator must confirm asystole in more than one lead. When using a monitor/defibrillator, the axis of the paddles can be moved 90° as from lead II to MCL1.

Once "true asystole" has been determined, treatment must proceed according to the sequence outlined in the asystole algorithm (Figure 10–8).

- **STEP 1:**
  Continue CPR
  Intubate at once
  Obtain IV access
  Confirm asystole in more than one lead

- **STEP 2:** Consider possible treatable causes
  Hypoxia
  Hyperkalemia
  Hypokalemia
  Pre-existing acidosis
  Drug overdose
  Hypothermia

Finding a treatable cause of asystole is the exception, rather than the rule. The team leader must conduct this search rapidly and aggresively. Fundamentals such as hyperventilation with oxygen and adequate chest compressions should always be given highest priority. Similarly, narcotic reversal, when indicated, can produce a dramatic recovery. It is helpful to note that naloxone can be administered endotracheally.

Asystole Treatment Algorithm

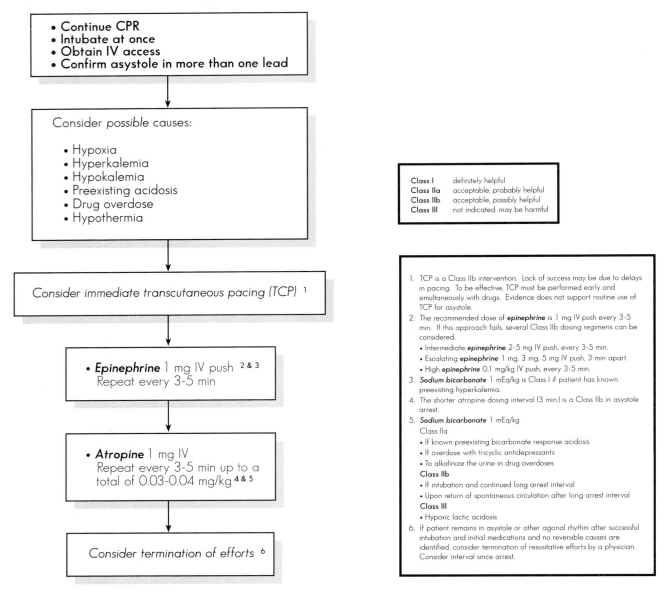

Figure 10–8. The asystole algorithm. "False asystole" is usually the result of operator error. "True asystole" usually represents a terminal event and is rarely the result of a treatable underlying cause. (Algorithm copyright 1992, American Medical Association; JAMA, October 28, 1992; pp 2199–2241.)

- **STEP 3:** Consider transcutaneous pacing

    The routine use of TCP in asystole is discouraged. The guidelines state that to be effective, TCP must be performed early and concurrently with drugs. Not surprisingly, the best time to initiate TCP is *prior* to pulselessness and asystole.

- **STEP 4:** Epinephrine 1.0 mg IV push. Repeat every 3 to 5 min.

  One of epinephrine's pharmacologic actions is its ability to restore spontaneous contractions in asystole.

- **STEP 5:** Atropine 1.0 mg IV push. Repeat every 3 to 5 min up to a maximum dose of 0.04 mg/kg (3.0 mg for a 70-kg victim).

  Atropine is part of the generalized therapeutic interventions recommended for cardiac arrest not associated with VF/VT or other tachyarrhythmias.

  Administration of atropine more frequently than every 3 to 5 minutes is considered a class IIb (possibly helpful) intervention.

Examples of Asystole

Depicted below are several examples of asystole. Figure 10–9 shows ventricular, but not atrial asystole. In Figure 10–10, the development of both ventricular and atrial asystole can be noted. Figure 10–11 also shows the onset of complete asystole.

PULSELESS ELECTRICAL ACTIVITY (PEA)

Definition

PEA is defined by the existence of an ECG other than VF/VT and a pulse that cannot be detected by *palpation* or *sphygmomanometry*.

At the top of the PEA algorithm (Figure 10–12) and below is a listing of the arrhythmias associated with PEA:

- Electromechanical dissociation (EMD)
- Pseudo-EMD
- Idioventricular and ventricular escape rhythms
- Bradyasystolic and agonal rhythms
- Postdefibrillation ideoventricular rhythms

Clinicians traditionally use the term *electromechanical dissociation* (EMD) when pulselessness exists despite a normal QRS complex.

EMD is a state in which organized electrical depolarization occurs throughout the ventricular muscle mass. Despite normal conduction, contraction of myofibrils is thought to *not* take place. As a result, cardiac output ceases and the victim becomes pulseless.

More recently, research on patients with clinical signs of EMD has been conducted using indwelling aortic catheters. These studies have revealed that pressure gradients synchronous with ventricular depolarization, and hence myocardial contraction, *can* exist during EMD.

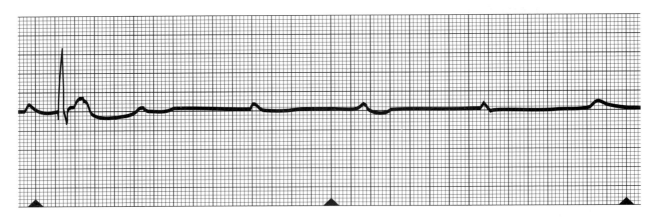

Figure 10–9. Onset of ventricular asystole with persistent atrial activity. In this electrocardiogram, a normal QRS-T originating in the sinus node is followed by ventricular asystole. P waves occurring at a rate of about 50/min are subsequently not conducted.

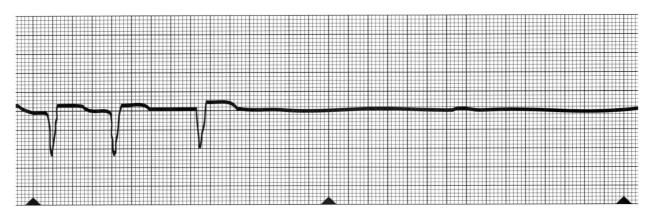

Figure 10–10. Onset of asystole. After three isolated ideoventricular complexes, atrial and ventricular asystole are noted.

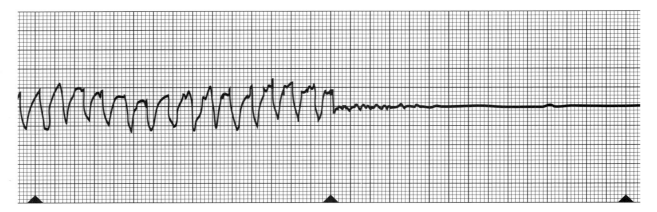

Figure 10–11. Abrupt onset of asystole. In this ECG, asystole develops precipitously during a run of VF/VT. Typically, the ECG undergoes gradual changes from VT to coarse VF and then to fine VF, before progressing to asystole.

Pulseless Electrical Activity (PEA) Algorithm
(Electromechanical Dissociation [EMD])

Includes:

- Electromechanical dissociation (EMD)
- Pseudo EMD
- Idioventricular rhythms
- Ventricular escape rhythms
- Bradyasystolic rhythms
- Post defibrillation idioventricular rhythms

- Continue CPR
- Intubate at once
- Obtain IV access
- Assess blood flow using Doppler ultrasound, end tidal CO_2, Electrocardiography or arterial line

---

Consider *possible* causes:

- Hypovolemia (volume infusion)
- Hypoxia (ventilation)
- Cardiac tamponade (pericardiocentesis)
- Tension pneumothorax (needle decompression)
- Hypothermia (see hypothermia algorithm)
- Massive pulmonary embolism (surgery, *thrombolytics*)

- Drug overdoses such as tricyclics, digitalis, β blockers, calcium channel blockers
- Hyperkalemia [1]
- Acidosis [2]
- Massive acute myocardial infarction

Note: Possible therapies and treatments are given in parentheses

---

Class I   definitely helpful
Class IIa   acceptable, *probably* helpful
Class IIb   acceptable, *possibly* helpful
Class III   not indicated, may be harmful

---

1. *Sodium bicarbonate* 1 mEq/kg is Class I if patient has known preexisting hyperkalemia.
2. *Sodium bicarbonate* 1 mEq/kg
   Class IIa
   - If known preexisting bicarbonate-responsive acidosis
   - If overdose with tricyclic antidepressants
   - To alkalinize the urine in drug overdoses
   Class IIb
   - If intubation and continued long arrest interval
   - Upon return of spontaneous circulation after long arrest interval
   Class III
   - Hypoxic lactic acidosis
3. The recommended dose of *epinephrine* is 1 mg IV push every 3-5 min. If this approach fails, several Class IIb dosing regimens can be considered.
   - Intermediate *epinephrine* 2-5 mg IV push, every 3-5 min.
   - Escalating *epinephrine* 1 mg, 3 mg, 5 mg IV push, 3 min. apart.
   - High *epinephrine* 0.1 mg/kg IV push, every 3-5 min.
4. The shorter atropine dosing interval (3 min.) is *possibly* helpful in cardiac arrest (Class IIb).

- *Epinephrine* 1 mg IV push [3]
  Repeat every 3-5 min

- If absolute bradycardia (<60 BPM) or relative bradycardia, give atropine 1 mg IV
- Repeat every 3-5 min to a total of 0.03-0.04 mg/kg [4]

Figure 10–12. The pulseless electrical activity (PEA) algorithm. PEA is defined as the presence of pulselessness despite the appearance of electrical activity other than VF or VT. In contrast to asystole, PEA is often the result of a treatable underlying cause. (Algorithm copyright 1992, American Medical Association; JAMA, October 28, 1992; pp 2199–2241.)

This has led to the adoption of the term *pseudo-EMD*. This term is meant to describe the following clinical situation:

- A pulse cannot be detected by palpation or sphygmomanometry.
- An essentially normal QRS complex.
- Some evidence of cardiac output exists as a result of:
    Doppler ultrasound
    Echocardiography
    Systemic arterial catheterization
    End tidal CO_2 monitoring

Examples of Narrow-complex PEA

Figure 10–13 illustrates narrow-complex arrhythmias associated with EMD/pseudo-EMD. Although these examples are bradyarrhythmias, PEA/EMD often presents as a rhythm with a rate greater than 60/min.

PEA is not an arrhythmia; it is a clinical situation. Reflecting this fact, the AHA *Instructor's Manual for ACLS* suggests using a "rhythm" with a rate of 100/min to represent *all* etiologies of PEA.

Examples of Wide-complex PEA

Figures 10–14, 10–15, and 10–16 illustrate broad-complex PEAs. Among them are:

- Idioventricular and ventricular escape rhythms
- Bradyasystolic and agonal rhythms

These wide-complex rhythms have been identified as causes of PEA. The JAMA guidelines refer to several studies that associate these particular arrhythmias with unfavorable outcomes. Additionally, these arrhythmias may be seen following *massive acute myocardial infarction*. Thus, their presence, like that of asystole, can represent confirmation of death.

There is a long list of agents that can result in wide-complex PEA when overdosage exists. Among them are:

- Digitalis
- Beta blockers
- Calcium channel blockers
- Tricyclic antidepressants

In these instances, prompt intervention with drug specific therapy is necessary.

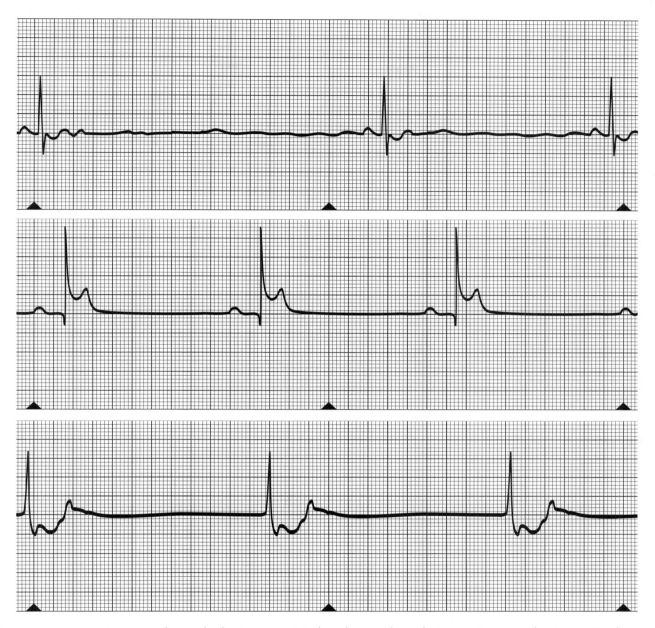

Figure 10–13. Narrow complex arrhythmias associated with EMD/pseudo-EMD. Because the top ECG does not demonstrate any markers of ischemia or injury, it is typical of pulselessness due to a nonischemic event. The ECG on the bottom is a junctional bradycardia with a rate of 23/min. The absence of sinus node activity is not a favorable prognostic marker.

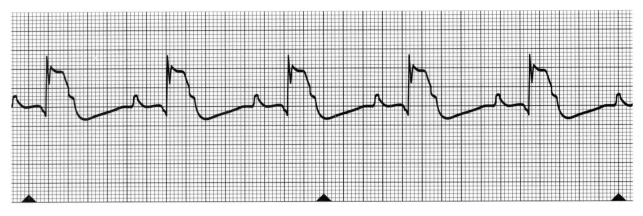

Figure 10–14. Broad-complex PEA with atrial activity. This strip demonstrates a broad QRS-T complex with a highly elevated ST segment. This is characteristic of severe myocardial injury.

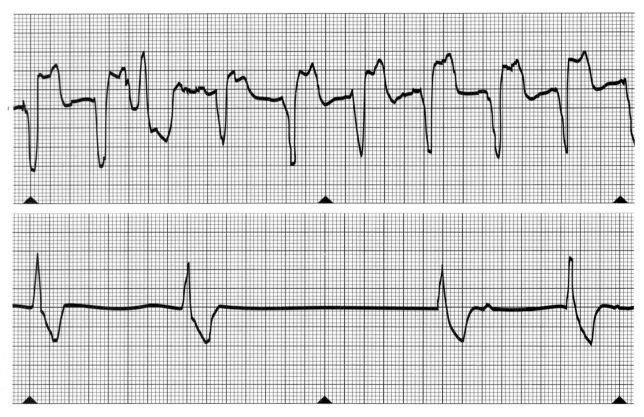

Figure 10–15. Idioventricular complexes are characteristically broad and monomorphic. The top ECG is an accelerated idioventricular rhythm so named because the rate is *greater* than 40/min. The bottom strip represents an idioventricular escape rhythm with characteristic escape rate of *less* than 40/min. Both are associated with poor outcomes unless they are due to a treatable underlying cause.

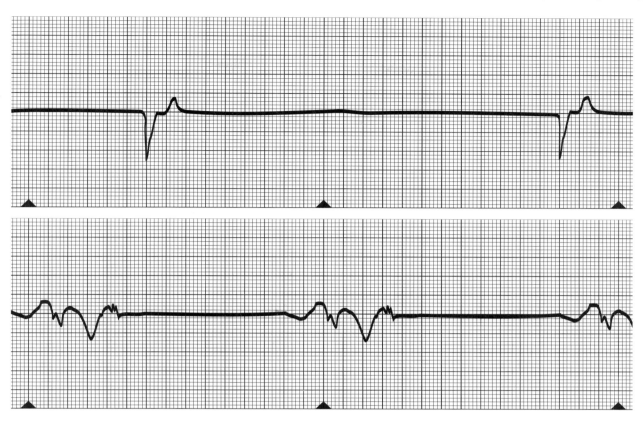

Figure 10–16. Bradyasystolic and agonal rhythms. The occasional bradyasystolic ventricular escape complex seen in the top ECG strip is generally considered a terminal event. The slurred agonal "rhythm" is also viewed as end-stage electrical activity.

Treatment of PEA

In direct contradistinction to asystole, when cardiac arrest is due to PEA, a treatable underlying cause is often responsible.

Therefore, the ACLS provider when confronted with PEA must immediately begin searching for a treatable underlying cause.

Below and in the PEA algorithm (Figure 10–12) is a list of possible causes of PEA. Next to each cause in parentheses are possible treatments or therapies.

- Hypovolemia (volume infusion)
- Hypoxia (ventilation)
- Cardiac tamponade (pericardiocentesis)
- Tension pneumothorax (needle decompression)
- Hypothermia (see hypothermia algorithm, section IV)
- Massive pulmonary embolism (surgery, thrombolytics)
- Drug overdoses such as tricyclics, digitalis, beta blockers, calcium channel blockers

- Hyperkalemia (sodium bicarbonate is class I)
- Acidosis
- Massive acute myocardial infarction

In viewing this list, please note that the most common causes are stated at the top.

Nonspecific Therapeutic Interventions

- **Fluid Challenge.** Hypovolemia is the most common cause of PEA. It is also the easiest cause to treat. Therefore, it is wise to begin the search for treatable underlying causes with hypovolemia. Clues include:
  - Flat neck veins
  - History of fluid loss from GI system
  - Obvious trauma/bleeding
  - Doppler-detectable blood flow
- **Intubation and ventilation with 100% oxygen.** Because hypoventilation and hypoxemia are frequent causes of PEA, aggressive attention to the airway and ventilatory needs of the patient is always a top priority.

Pharmacologic Interventions

- **Epinephrine.** 1.0 mg IV push every 3 to 5 minutes. Epinephrine is the only class I agent for all forms of cardiac arrest.
- **Atropine.** 1.0 mg IV push every 3 to 5 minutes up to a total of 0.04 mg/kg. Atropine is indicated in PEAs that involve cardiac rates less than 60/min.

ELECTROCARDIOGRAPHIC ARTIFACT

The discussion of lethal arrhythmias must be rounded out by emphasizing that both asystole and VF/VT can be mimicked by oscilloscopic and electrocardiographic artifact. The worst case scenario would be administration of countershock to a patient in whom it is not indicated.

Examples of Artifact Relevant to ACLS

Illustrated below are examples of electrocardiographic artifact with which the ACLS provider should be familiar. First, when confronted with an isoelectric line on the ECG monitor (Figures 10–17 and 10–18) providers must immediately rule out "false asystole." This situation is frequently the result of a poor electrical connection.

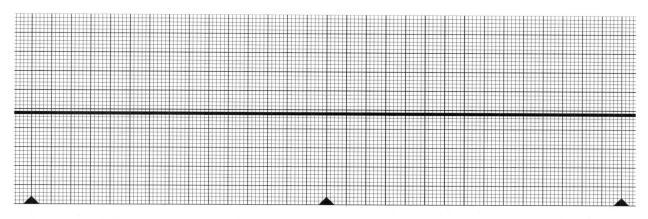

Figure 10–17. Lead disconnect or power failure artifact. A completely isoelectric line is almost always "false asystole." Leads or electrodes that are completely disconnected are the most common cause.

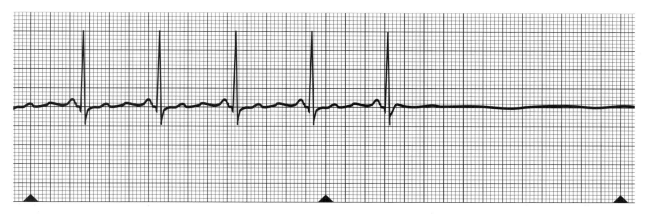

Figure 10–18. Loose electrode artifact. Loose skin-to-electrode contact is an extremely common occurrence. It can be caused by loosening of the electrode pad itself, by profuse diaphoresis, or by a loose electrode wire.

VF/VT can also be mimicked by ECG artifact as shown in Figures 10–19 and 10–20. Movement of large upper extremity muscles can produce substantial electronic noise. This is particularly true if ECG electrodes have been placed over a bony prominence such as the clavicle.

Figures 10–21 and 10–22 depict examples of high-frequency artifact such as can result from shivering, transport vehicle artifact, and from leakage of alternating current from electrical devices. Finally, Figure 10–23 shows the wandering baseline artifact typical of chest wall movement.

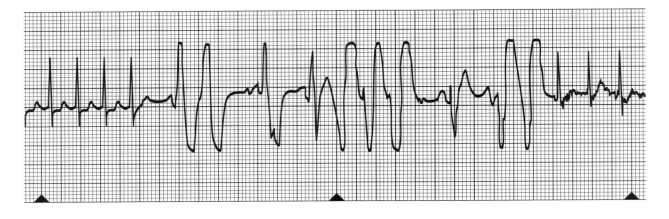

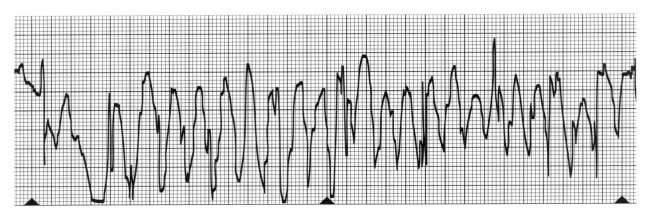

Figure 10–19. Shoulder movement in patient with electrode placement on the clavicles. Upper extremity movement by a patient whose electrodes have been placed over a bony prominence is a potentially dangerous combination in that VF/VT can be mimicked. Remember, "treat the patient, *not* the monitor."

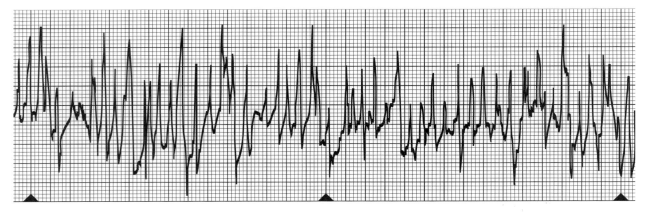

Figure 10–20. Large muscle tremor artifact. Seizure activity involves large skeletal muscles and can yield high amplitude high frequency artifact on the ECG. Because it also can mimic VF/VT, this is another potentially dangerous situation.

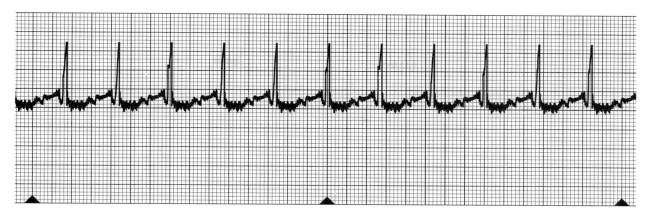

Figure 10–21. Transport vehicle and shivering artifact. High frequency, low amplitude artifact can be caused by fine muscle tremor. It can also be caused by ambulance movement. If the R–R interval were irregular, this could resemble atrial fibrillation and prompt unnecessary intervention.

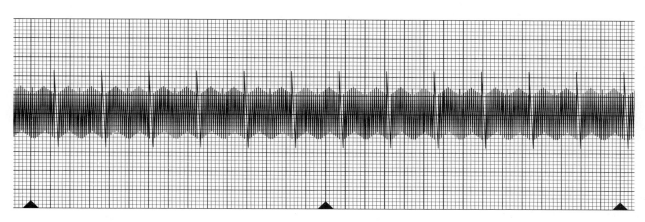

Figure 10–22. 60-cycle interference artifact. External power sources can leak enough electrical current to interfere with the ECG tracing. Electrical shavers and battery-powered devices are common culprits.

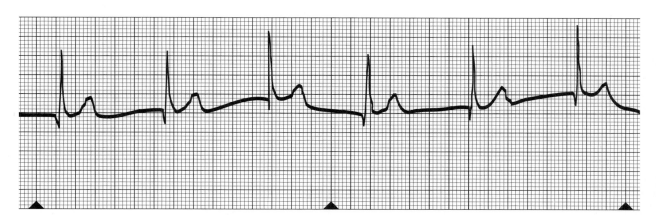

Figure 10–23. Respiratory artifact. Chest wall movement can cause the isoelectric baseline to wander. This distraction can be minimized by not placing electrodes over the lower ribs where chest wall movement is exaggerated.

BIBLIOGRAPHY

1. American Heart Association. Emergency Cardiac Care Committee and Subcommittees. Guidelines for cardiopulmonary resuscitation and emergency cardiac care. JAMA 1992;268:2171–2295
2. American Heart Association. Textbook of advanced cardiac life support. Dallas, TX: American Heart Association, 1994
3. American Heart Association. Instructor's manual for advanced cardiac life support. Dallas, TX: American Heart Association, 1994
4. Aufderheide TP, Thakur RK, Stueven HA, Aprahamian C, Zhu YR, Turk D, et al. Electrocardiographic characteristics in EMD. Resuscitation 1989;17:183–193
5. Bocka JJ, Overton DT, Hauser A. Electromechanical dissociation in human beings: en echocardiographic evaluation. Ann Emerg Med 1988;17:450–452
6. Bonnin M, Pepe P, Kimball K, Clark P. Distinct criteria for terminating resuscitation in the out of hospital setting. JAMA 1993;270:1457–1462
7. Hamill RJ. Resuscitation: when is enough enough? Respir Care 1995;40:515–527
8. Paradis NA, Martin GB, Goetting MG, et al. Aortic pressure during human cardiac arrest. Chest 1992;101:123–128
9. Robinson G, Hess D. Postdischarge survival and functional status following in-hospital CPR. Chest 1994;105:991–996
10. Rubenfield GD. Do not resuscitate orders: A critical review of the literature. Respir Care 1995;40:528–537
11. Stueven HA, Aufderheide T, Waite EM, Mateer JR. Electromechanical dissociation: six years prehospital experience. Resuscitation 1989;17:173–182

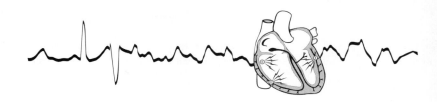

11. The Bradycardias

STABLE VERSUS UNSTABLE BRADYCARDIAS

Recommendations for management of excessively slow cardiac rhythms are summarized in the bradycardia algorithm (Figure 11–1).

This critical pathway begins with determination of the presence of an *absolute* or a *relative* bradycardia. For example, even though a patient whose heart rate is 65/min does not meet the strict definition of bradycardia, if they have serious signs and symptoms related to their slow heart rate, they are to be treated according to this algorithm.

The JAMA guidelines repeatedly remind us to "treat the patient, not the monitor." Thus, the algorithm next asks that the ACLS provider determine the presence or absence of hemodynamic stability.

The guidelines and the algorithm define hemodynamic instability as

Bradycardia Algorithm
(Patient is not in cardiac arrest)

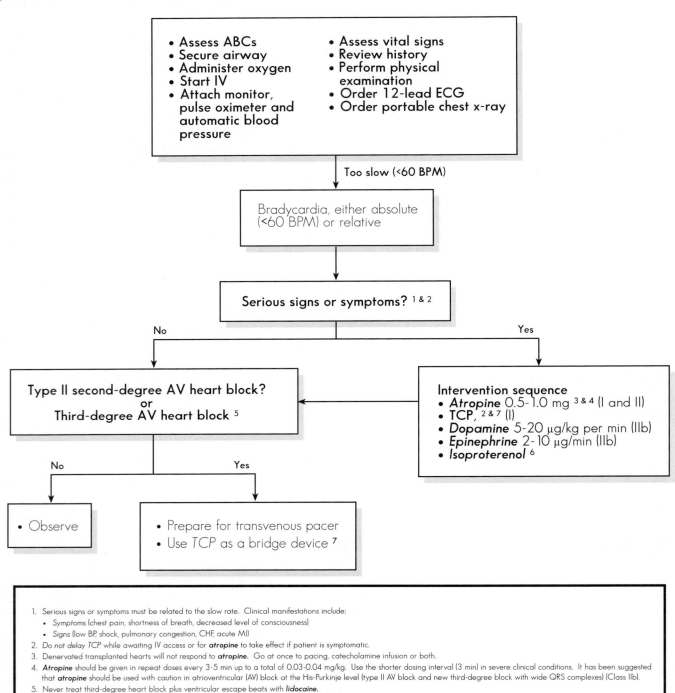

Figure 11–1. The bradycardia algorithm. This critical pathway is assessed in Case 7, Bradycardia. (Algorithm copyright 1992, American Medical Association; JAMA, October 28, 1992; pp 2199–2241.)

the presence of more than one of the following signs and symptoms, which *must be related to the slow rate itself.*

- *Signs* include:
    Chest pain
    Shortness of breath
    Decreased level of consciousness
- *Symptoms* include:
    Systolic BP less than 80 mm Hg
    Pulmonary congestion
    Peripheral hypoperfusion
    AMI

ESSENTIAL ACLS CURRICULA

The AHA *Instructor's Manual for ACLS* states that the following bradycardias should be part of an essential ACLS provider course:

- Sinus bradycardia
- Junctional rhythms
- First-degree AV block
- Second-degree type I AV block
- Second-degree type II AV block
- Third-degree AV block

SINUS BRADYCARDIA

ECG Appearance

As illustrated in Figure 11–2, sinus bradycardia is described as a monotonously regular succession of PQRS and T waves occurring at a rate less than 60/min.

- P waves are normally shaped and upright in leads I, II, and AVF. They are followed by a QRS complex.
- Conduction is normal. Thus, the PR interval is between 0.10 and 0.20 second and the QRS is between 0.04 and 0.12 second.

Causes

- Severe hypoxia
- Infarct/injury to the sinus node
- Vagal stimulation
- Digitalis
- Calcium channel blockers
- Beta-blocking agents

Significance in ACLS

This arrhythmia is a very common cause of hemodynamic instability. It is also the initial ECG noted in many patients who develop PEA.

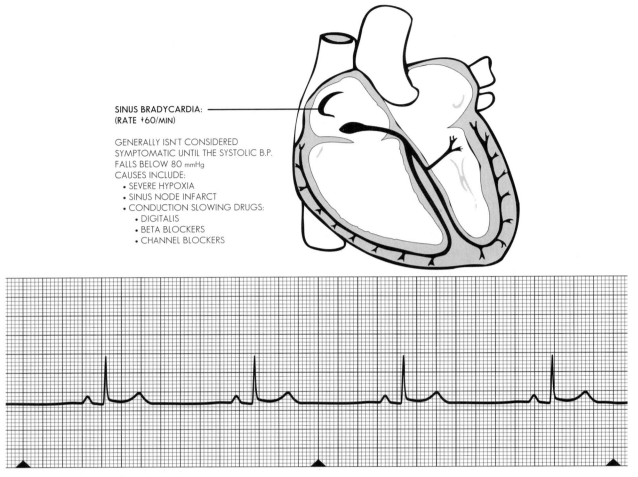

SINUS BRADYCARDIA:
(RATE ↓60/MIN)

GENERALLY ISN'T CONSIDERED
SYMPTOMATIC UNTIL THE SYSTOLIC B.P.
FALLS BELOW 80 mmHg
CAUSES INCLUDE:
• SEVERE HYPOXIA
• SINUS NODE INFARCT
• CONDUCTION SLOWING DRUGS:
  • DIGITALIS
  • BETA BLOCKERS
  • CHANNEL BLOCKERS

Figure 11–2. Sinus bradycardia is defined as a monotonously regular succession of PQRS and T waves occurring at a rate less than 60 min. Treatment generally is not required until the systolic BP falls below 80 mm Hg.

ACLS Intervention Sequence

Treatment is not required unless hemodynamic instability exists. The following intervention sequence is recommended in the bradycardia algorithm:

- Atropine 0.5 to 1.0 mg IV push. May be repeated every 3 to 5 min up to a maximum dose of 0.04 mg/kg
- Transcutaneous pacing if available (class I)
- Dopamine 5 to 20 µg/kg/min (class IIb)
- Epinephrine 2 to 10 µg/min (class IIb)
- Isoproterenol 2 to 10 µg/min (class IIb in low doses; class III at higher doses)

Examples of Sinus Bradycardia

Pictured below are several examples of sinus bradycardia. Figure 11–3 shows a narrow complex rhythm with a rate of 33/min. Figure 11–4 illustrates a sinus rhythm with a rate of 50/min. In the setting of ACLS its profoundly elevated ST segment would be an indication for a 12-lead ECG to

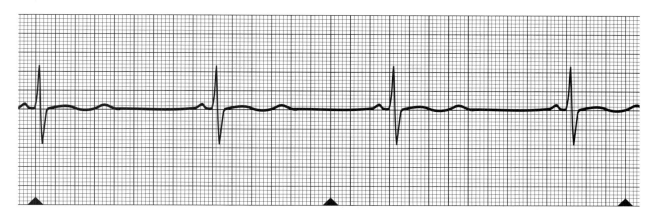

Figure 11–3. Sinus bradycardia with prominent U wave. Very slow sinus bradycardias are often associated with hypotension despite the absence of inverted T waves and elevated ST segments. The U wave is often a marker of hypokalemia.

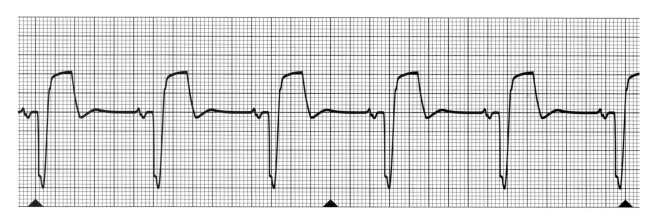

Figure 11–4. Sinus bradycardia with marked ST segment elevation. In the setting of ACLS and possible AMI, a patient presenting with this arrhythmia should be evaluated for thrombolytic therapy. Please refer to the discussion of the AMI algorithm in Chapter 9.

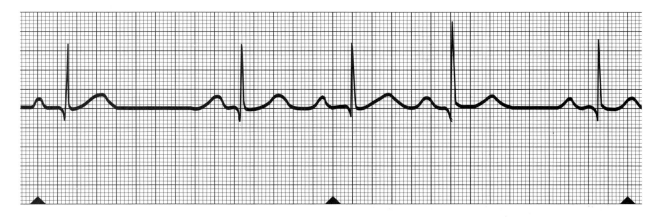

Figure 11–5. Sinus arrhythmia. This irregular rhythm appears to be a sinus bradycardia, but the rate is actually 68/min. Sinus arrhythmia is a normal irregularity often seen in the physically fit and in younger patients. In these individuals, changes in vagal tone occur synchronously with ventilatory efforts. The result is periodic speeding and slowing of sinus node impulse formation.

help determine the need for thrombolytic therapy. Sinus arrhythmia, shown in Figure 11–5, though common and asymptomatic must be considered in the differential of bradycardias.

JUNCTIONAL RHYTHMS

So-called junctional escape pacemaker cells are located in the AV node and in the bundle of His. These cells have an inherent rate of 40 to 60 min.

Because of their location, impulses generated by these tissues must travel cephalad to discharge the atria. This results in P waves that are *inverted* in leads II and III.

As depicted in Figure 11–6, depending on the site of origin of the impulse, the inverted P wave can precede, be buried in, or *follow* the QRS complex. In the latter event, the ectopic focus is located so close to the bundle branches that ventricular depolarization actually occurs prior to that of the atria.

Because these arrhythmias are supraventricular in origin, the QRS complexes are of normal width.

Causes of Junctional Rhythms

Sinus Pause or Sinus Arrest

Because junctional tissues have an inherent rate of 40 to 60/min should sinus impulse formation fall *below* this rate, a junctional pacemaker can initiate an escape beat. An example of a *junctional escape complex* is seen in Figure 11–7.

Should *sinus arrest* occur, a junctional escape focus may take complete responsibility for discharging the ventricles. The result is called a *junctional rhythm.* These typically have a rate of 40 to 60/min. An example of a junctional rhythm is seen in Figure 11–8.

Accelerated Junctional Tissue Automaticity

Accelerated junctional tissue automaticity is usually the result of an ischemic event. It can also be secondary to digitalis overadministration. *Premature junctional contractions* (PJCs) are the result of an irritable junctional focus that fires early for the dominant rhythm. The compensatory pause following a PJC can be either complete or incomplete. Figure 11–9 shows a PJC with an incomplete compensatory pause.

When a junctional ectopic focus initiates rhythm at a rate greater than 100/min, it is termed a *junctional tachycardia.* Figure 11–10 is an example of junctional tachycardia in a patient with severe chest pain.

When a junctional focus results in a rhythm with a rate of 60 to 100/min, it is called an *accelerated junctional rhythm.* Figure 11–11 shows an accelerated junctional rhythm with a rate of approximately 70/min.

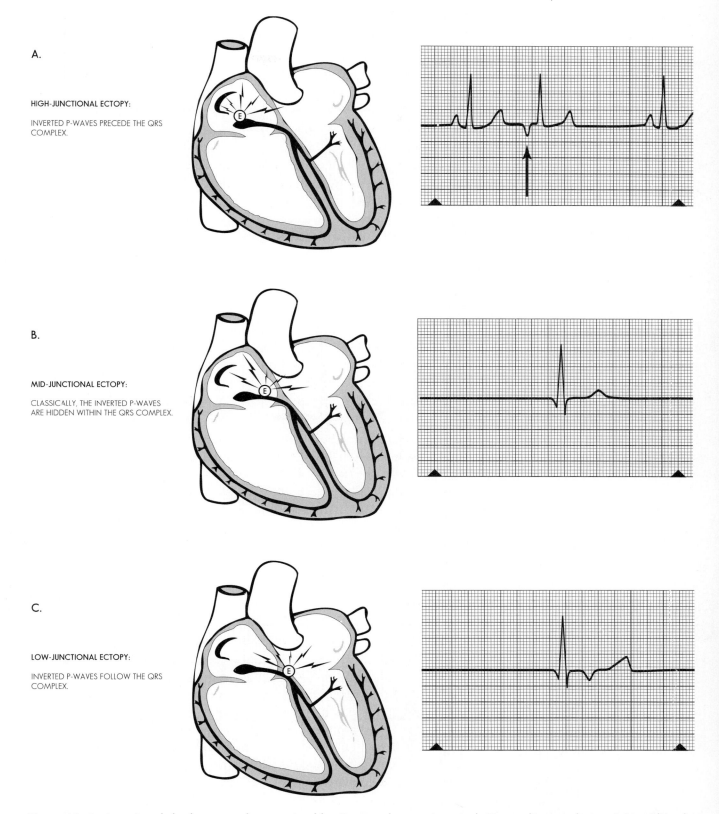

A.

HIGH-JUNCTIONAL ECTOPY:

INVERTED P-WAVES PRECEDE THE QRS
COMPLEX.

B.

MID-JUNCTIONAL ECTOPY:

CLASSICALLY, THE INVERTED P-WAVES
ARE HIDDEN WITHIN THE QRS COMPLEX.

C.

LOW-JUNCTIONAL ECTOPY:

INVERTED P-WAVES FOLLOW THE QRS
COMPLEX.

Figure 11–6. Junctional rhythms are characterized by P wave that are inverted. Depending on their origin within the AV junction, these P waves can either precede, be buried in, or follow the QRS complex.

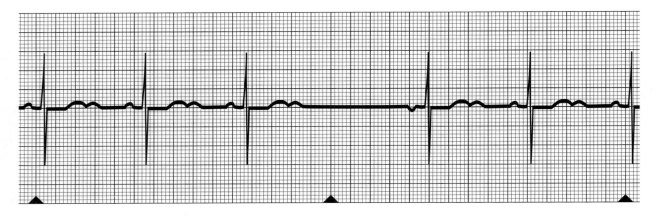

Figure 11–7. A junctional escape beat is initiated following a sinus pause.

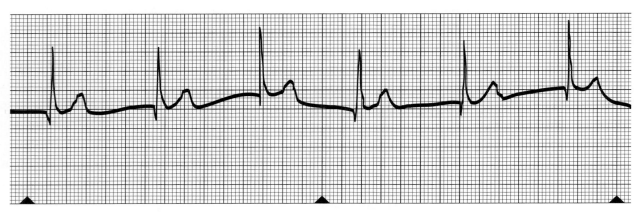

Figure 11–8. Junctional rhythm with a rate of approximately 60/min.

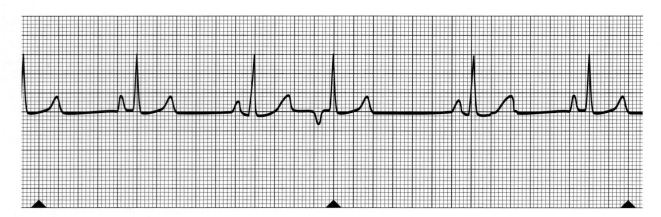

Figure 11–9. Premature junctional contraction with an incomplete compensatory pause.

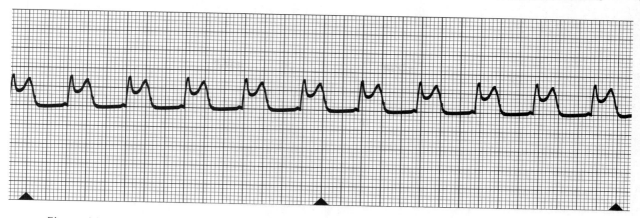

Figure 11–10. Junctional tachycardia (rate is 103/min) with considerable ST segment elevation.

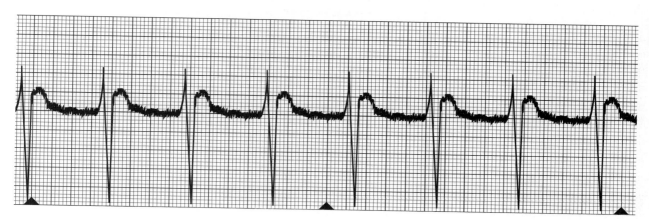

Figure 11–11. Accelerated junctional rhythm with 60 cycle artifact.

FIRST- AND SECOND-DEGREE TYPE I AV BLOCKS

Significance in ACLS

First- and second-degree type I AV blocks are most commonly the result of block at the level of the AV node. This *nodal block pattern* depicted in Figure 11–12 is often the result of drugs, *not* an ischemic event.

Agents that have a negative dromotropic effect are most frequently implicated. Conduction-slowing drugs include:

- Digitalis
- Calcium channel blockers
- Beta blockers

Because the block does *not* involve the bundle branches, the QRS complexes are usually of normal width. Correspondingly, the majority of patients with these arrhythmias are hemodynamically stable. With few dropped

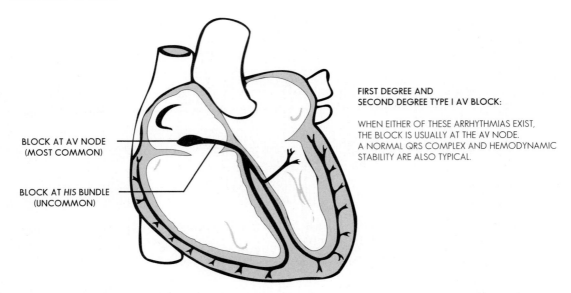

FIRST DEGREE AND
SECOND DEGREE TYPE I AV BLOCK:

WHEN EITHER OF THESE ARRHYTHMIAS EXIST,
THE BLOCK IS USUALLY AT THE AV NODE.
A NORMAL QRS COMPLEX AND HEMODYNAMIC
STABILITY ARE ALSO TYPICAL.

BLOCK AT AV NODE
(MOST COMMON)

BLOCK AT *HIS* BUNDLE
(UNCOMMON)

Figure 11–12. *Nodal* AV block pattern for first- and second-degree type I AV blocks. When conduction delay is in or near the AV node, these two arrhythmias often result. Because the bundle branches are not involved, the resulting QRS complex is usually normal. Correspondingly hemodynamic instability is rare.

beats and with normal ventricular conduction, it is rare for these arrhythmias to cause systemic hypotension or pulmonary congestion.

ECG Appearance

First-degree AV Block

In first-degree AV block *all* P waves are conducted and thus are followed by a normal QRS complex.

The abnormality in first-degree AV block is *slowing* of conduction through the AV node. Thus, the primary ECG manifestation is a PR interval greater than 0.20 second.

Essentially, first-degree AV block is a sinus rhythm with a widened PR interval. Figure 11–13 shows examples of first degree AV block.

Second-degree Type I AV Block

The criteria for this arrhythmia is progressive widening of the PR interval followed by dropping of a P wave.

This arrhythmia is a regular irregularity. That is, it has a cycle that repeats itself. A common pattern is two conducted beats followed by a nonconducted impulse. This is referred to as a 3:2 conduction ratio. 4:3 and 2:1 presentation are also common. It is not unusual for patients with this arrhythmia to change patterns over the course of time. For example, as the

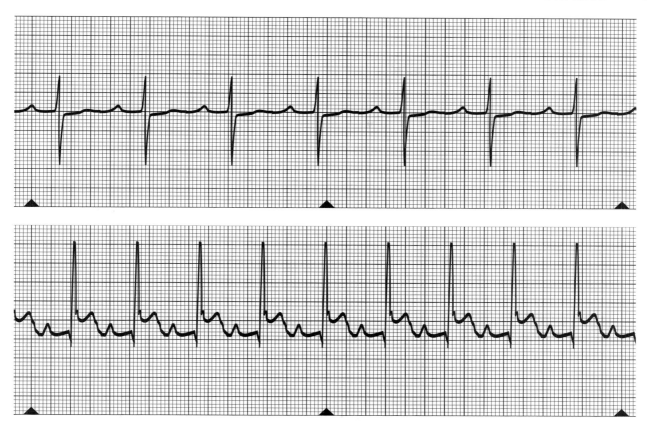

Figure 11–13. Examples of first-degree AV block. The top ECG is a normal sinus rhythm (NSR) with a rate of 70/min and a PR interval of 0.30 sec. The bottom strip is also an NSR. This time, the rate is 90/min and the PR interval is again approximately 0.30 second.

underlying cause of the arrhythmia responds to therapy, fewer beats tend to be dropped. Correspondingly, the pattern might change from 2:1 to 4:3.

Figures 11–14 and 11–15 show examples of second-degree type I AV block with various conduction ratios.

ACLS Intervention Sequence

Patients with first- and second-degree type I AV block are rarely unstable. Nonspecific interventions include:

- Monitoring
- Lowering blood levels of digitalis, beta blockers, and calcium channel blockers by tapering or by targeted therapy.

Should severe signs and symptoms be present, ALCS providers should recommend the following intervention sequence from the bradycardia algorithm:

- Atropine 0.5 to 1.0 mg (classes I and IIa)
- Transcutaneous pacing if available (class I)
- Dopamine 5 to 20 μg/min (class IIb)
- Epinephrine 2 to 10 μg/min (class IIb)
- Isoproterenol 2 to 10 μg/min (class IIb in low doses; class III at higher doses)

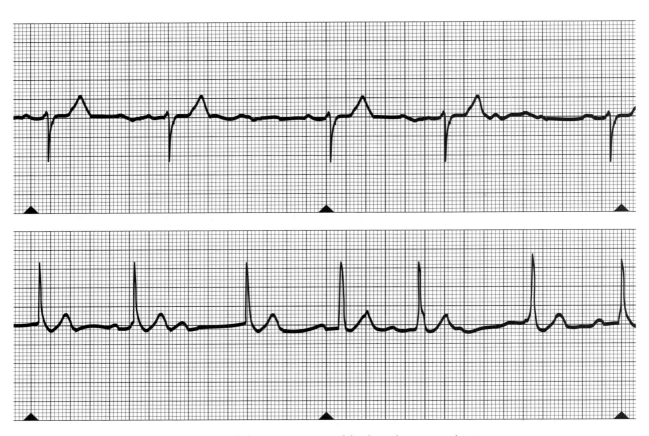

Figure 11–14. Second-degree type I AV block with 3:2 conduction pattern.

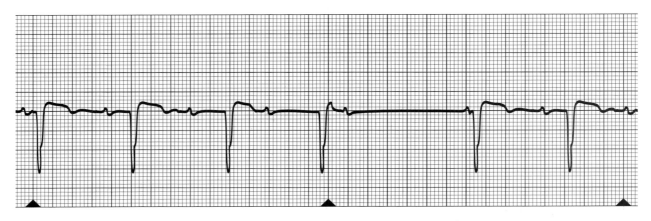

Figure 11–15. Second-degree type I AV block with 5:4 conduction pattern.

SECOND-DEGREE TYPE II AND THIRD-DEGREE AV BLOCKS

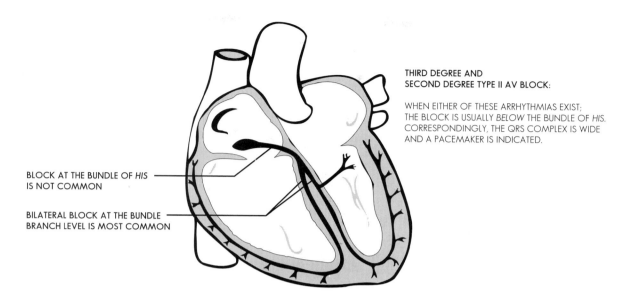

THIRD DEGREE AND
SECOND DEGREE TYPE II AV BLOCK:

WHEN EITHER OF THESE ARRHYTHMIAS EXIST;
THE BLOCK IS USUALLY *BELOW* THE BUNDLE OF *HIS*.
CORRESPONDINGLY, THE QRS COMPLEX IS WIDE
AND A PACEMAKER IS INDICATED.

BLOCK AT THE BUNDLE OF *HIS*
IS NOT COMMON

BILATERAL BLOCK AT THE BUNDLE
BRANCH LEVEL IS MOST COMMON

Figure 11–16. *Infranodal* AV block pattern for third-degree and second-degree type II AV blocks. When the block is at or near the bundle branch level, AMI is likely a cause, the prognosis is less favorable, and hemodynamic instability is common.

Significance in ACLS

Second-degree type II and third-degree AV blocks are most commonly the result of block at the bundle branch level. This *infranodal block pattern* (Figure 11–16) is usually the result of an ischemic event. It is rarely associated with drug effect. A common source of these arrhythmias is acute anteroseptal or anterior myocardial infarction.

When complete blockage exists in both bundle branches, as is the case with third-degree AV block, the ventricles must rely on ventricular escape foci with their inherent rate of less than 40/min. As a result, the QRS complexes will be wide and the patient is likely to be hemodynamically unstable.

In second-degree type II AV block, there is complete blockage of one bundle branch and intermittent block of the other branch. Dropped beats occur when both branches are blocked at the same time. Conducted beats will typically display a wide QRS because unilateral bundle branch block still exists.

ECG Appearance

Second-degree Type II AV Block

The ECG criteria for this arrhythmia is sudden dropping of impulses without gradual widening of the PR interval.

The PR interval may be within normal limits or it may be wide, but it typically does *not* change prior to dropped beats. A common example of second-degree type II AV block is the so-called "type II 2:1 AV block."

Here there are two P waves for every QRS complex. Figure 11–17 shows examples of type II 2:1 AV block.

It is common for second-degree type II AV block to progress to third-degree AV block. Before that occurs, type II 3:1 and 4:1 block patterns are often seen. Here two out of three or three of four P waves are blocked. An example is seen in Figure 11–18.

Third-degree AV Block

In third-degree AV block *all* P waves are blocked. This arrhythmia is called complete heart block because when both bundle branches are blocked, *supraventricular impulses are not conducted* to the ventricles.

As a result, the ventricles must be paced by ventricular escape pacemaker cells with their inherent rate of less than 40/min.

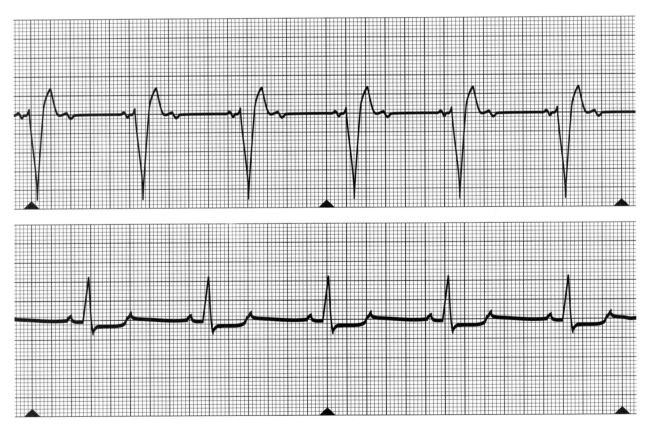

Figure 11–17. Examples of second-degree type II 2:1 AV block. Please note how these ECGs meet previously described criteria:
- Constant PR interval
- Wide QRS (the conducted beats are due to unilateral bundle branch block)
- Two P waves for each QRS (both bundle branches must be blocked for non-conduction to occur)

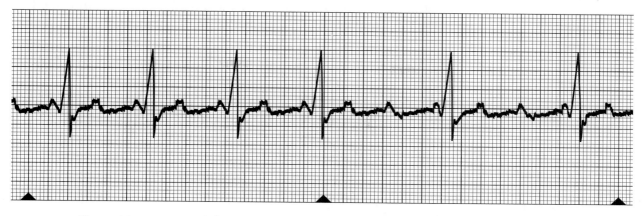

Figure 11–18. Second-degree type II 2:1 AV block progressing to a 3:1 block pattern.

Despite the absence of conduction, the sinus node typically continues to generate P waves at a rate of 60 to 100/min.

Thus, as displayed in Figure 11–19, the classic ECG criteria for third-degree AV block are:

- Atrial rate of 60 to 100/min.
- Ventricular rate of between 30 to 40/min.
- No relationship between atrial and ventricular activity. Because they are depolarized by different pacemakers at different rates, the P waves seem to "march" through the complexes.
- The QRS complexes are wide reflecting their ectopic origin.

Figure 11–20 contains other examples of third-degree AV block.

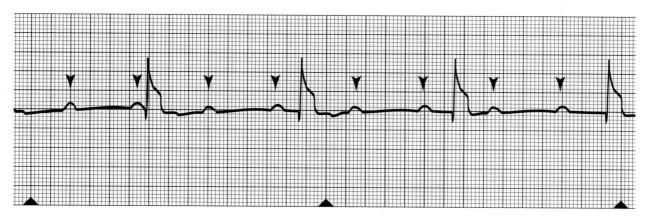

Figure 11–19. Example of third-degree AV block that meets "textbook" criteria. Note ECG of criteria that define third-degree block:
- Ventricular rate of 30 to 40/min
- Atrial rate of 60 to 100/min
- Wide QRS complexes
- P waves "marching" through the complexes

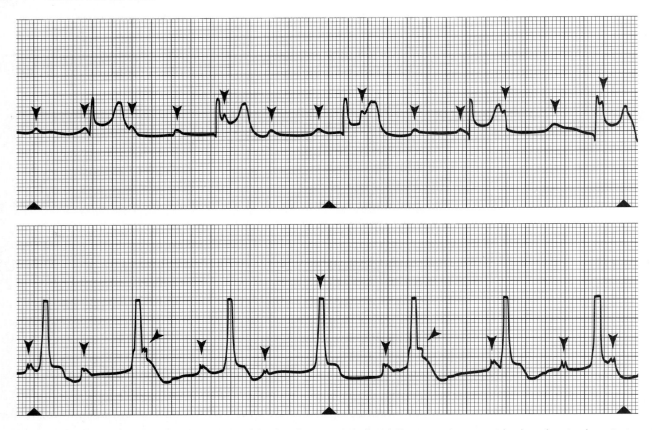

Figure 11–20. Examples of third-degree AV block. These examples fall somewhat outside the classic description. In the top strip, the atrial rate is a rapid 130/min. In the bottom ECG, the ventricular rate is 65/min. In both cases the QRS is widened, reflecting block at the bundle branch level and a ventricular escape rhythm. P waves are marked by arrows to show how they "march" in and out of the QRS–T complexes.

Occasionally, third-degree AV block may be caused by a nodal block. When this is the case, a junctional escape focus will discharge the ventricles. Predictably, the resultant complexes will occur at a rate of 40 to 60/min and be narrow. Figure 11–21 shows an example of third-degree AV block with a narrow QRS complex.

Like second-degree type I AV block, complete heart block caused by a nodal block is:

- Often drug-related and transient
- Not likely to cause serious signs and symptoms
- Not likely to require a transvenous pacemaker

ACLS Intervention Sequence

The JAMA guidelines state that second-degree type II and third-degree AV blocks are usually associated with hemodynamic instability, broad QRS complexes, and acute anterior or anteroseptal MI.

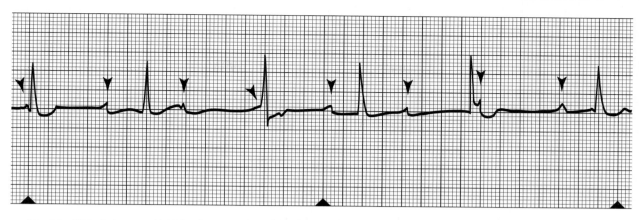

Figure 11–21. Third-degree AV block caused by block above the bundle branches. When complete heart block occurs above the bundle branches, a junctional escape pacemaker depolarizes the ventricles. Thus, patients are often hemodynamically stable and generally do not require a pacemaker.

When this is the case, the following intervention sequence is recommended:

- Prepare for a *transvenous* pacemaker.
- Use TCP as a bridging device.
- Use *atropine* until capture can be achieved with TCP.
- Prepare a standby dopamine or epinephrine drip should delays in pacing occur.
- Isoproterenol should only be used as a last resort.

The bradycardia algorithm states that atropine is a class IIb intervention when second-degree type II or third-degree AV block with wide QRS complexes exist. As such, it must be used with caution.

BIBLIOGRAPHY

1. American Heart Association. Emergency Cardiac Care Committee and Subcommittees. Guidelines for cardiopulmonary resuscitation and emergency cardiac care. JAMA 1992;268:2171–2295
2. American Heart Association. Textbook of advanced cardiac life support. Dallas, TX: American Heart Association, 1994
3. American Heart Association. Instructor's manual for advanced cardiac life support. Dallas, TX: American Heart Association, 1994
4. Gonzalez ER. Pharmacologic controversies in CPR. Ann Emerg Med 1993; 22(Part 2):317–323

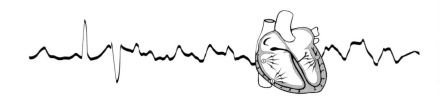

12. The Tachycardias

STABLE VERSUS UNSTABLE TACHYCARDIAS

Recommendations for management of rapid cardiac rhythms are summarized in the tachycardia and the electrical cardioversion algorithms (Figures 12–1 and 12–2).

A central focus of both pathways is determining whether the patient is hemodynamically stable or unstable.

In the setting of ACLS, tachycardias produce the same serious signs and symptoms as bradycardias. Were invasive hemodynamic measurements possible, these signs and symptoms would be marked by a cardiac index less than 2.2 L/min/M² and/or a pulmonary wedge pressure greater than 18 mm Hg.

In the absence of these measurements, the ACLS provider must make

Tachycardia Algorithm

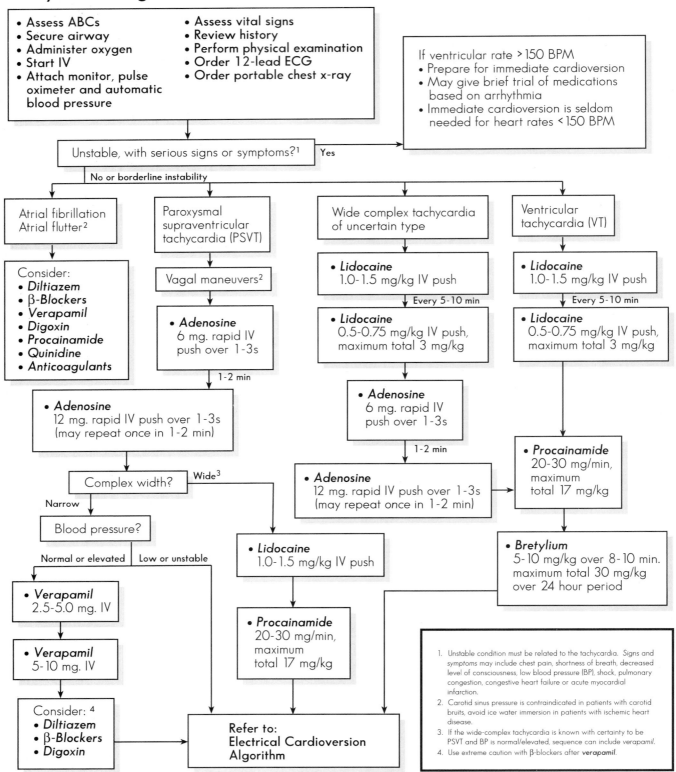

Figure 12–1. The stable tachycardia algorithm. Vital points emphasized in this algorithm are: (1) If the patient is unstable, prepare for immediate cardioversion. (2) Treat wide-complex tachycardias as if they were VT. (Algorithm copyright 1992, American Medical Association; JAMA, October 28, 1992; pp 2199–2241.)

Electrical Cardioversion/Unstable Tachycardia Algorithm
(Patient not in cardiac arrest)

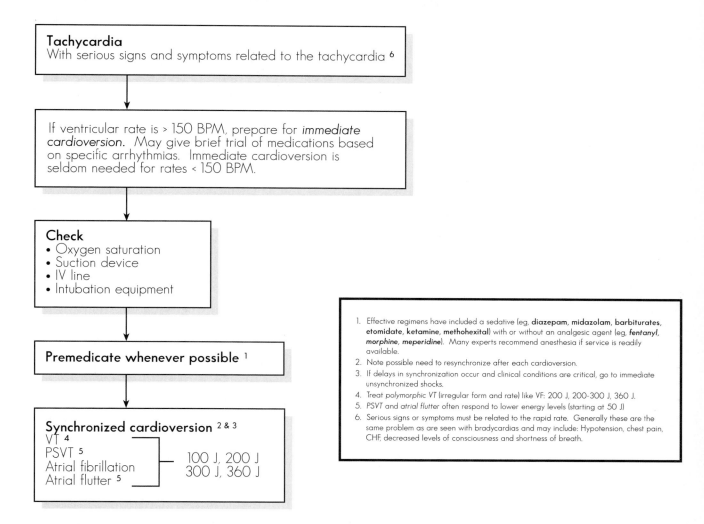

Figure 12–2. The unstable tachycardia algorithm. (Algorithm copyright 1992, American Medical Association; JAMA, October 28, 1992; pp 2199–2241.)

the determination of stability or instability by noting the presence of *more than one* of the following familiar signs and symptoms.

An important point emphasized in the algorithm is that serious signs and symptoms are *seldom* present at rates less than 150/min. Conversely, rates greater than this number may exist in the presence of hemodynamic stability:

- *Signs*
    Chest pain
    Shortness of breath
    Decreased level of consciousness

- *Symptoms*
  Systolic BP less than 80 mm Hg
  Pulmonary congestion
  Peripheral hypoperfusion
  AMI

The next question that must be answered is *not* an academic one. The ACLS provider must determine if the signs and symptoms are *caused* by the tachycardia or if the signs and symptoms are *causing* the rapid heart rate.

Consider the following self-study question: A patient is brought to the emergency room complaining of severe chest pain and shortness of breath. On physical examination, jugular venous distention is noted and bi-basal rales are heard on auscultation. The ECG reveals sinus tachycardia with frequent PVCs, and the BP is 130/85. Which of the following therapeutic agents is *least* advisable at the time?

A. Oxygen via mask
B. Morphine sulfate 1 to 3 mg IV
C. Nitroglycerin spray or sublingual
D. Lidocaine 1.0 to 1.5 mg/kg IV

Answer . . . D: Lidocaine is least clearly indicated at this time. Sinus tachycardia is not a rhythm to be treated. It is a healthy response to the need for increased oxygen transport. Similarly, the PVCs and the anginal pain are probably both the result of myocardial ischemia. Pain relief with morphine, improvement of hemodynamics with nitroglycerin, and increasing SaO_2 with oxygen are all aimed at the underlying cause. Their use is often rewarded with both improvement in symptoms and arrhythmia resolution.

ESSENTIAL ACLS CURRICULA

The AHA *Instructor's Manual for ACLS* states that the following tachycardias should be part of an essentials of ACLS provider course:

- Sinus tachycardia
- Atrial flutter
- Atrial fibrillation
- PSVT (including atrial tachycardia with block)
- Ventricular tachycardia (including Torsade de pointes)
- Wide-complex tachycardias of uncertain origin

You will note that all of these arrhythmias except sinus tachycardia are the result of *premature ectopy.* This fundamental principle is discussed in Chapter 8, Mechanisms of Arrhythmia Formation.

SINUS TACHYCARDIA

ECG Appearance

Sinus tachycardia is described as a monotonously regular succession of P–QRS–T waves occurring at a rate of greater than 100/min (Figure 12–3).

- P waves are normally shaped and upright in leads I, II, and AVF. They are followed by a QRS complex.
- Conduction is normal. Thus, the PR interval is between 0.10 and 0.20 second, and the QRS is between 0.04 and 0.12 seconds.
- *Distinct* P–QRS–T waves can usually be noted until rates exceed 160/min.

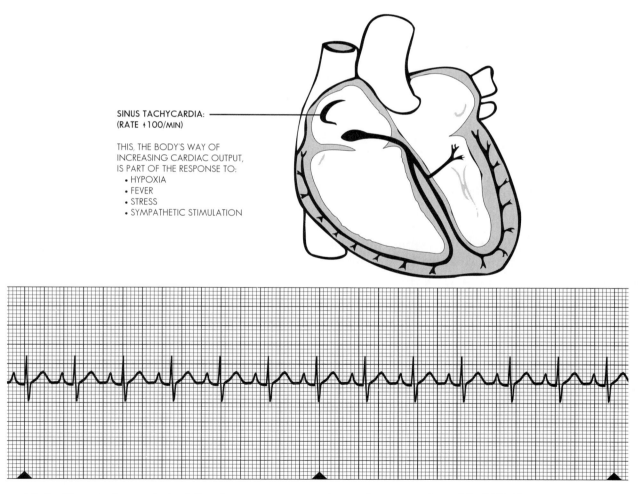

Figure 12–3. Sinus tachycardia is defined as a monotonously regular succession of P–QRS–T waves at a rate greater than 100/min. A healthy response to the need for oxygen transport, it does not represent an arrhythmia to be treated. Its presence is best thought of as a warning that an underlying problem exists.

Significance in ACLS

The organism's healthy response to sympathetic stimulation and the need for increased cardiac output, sinus tachycardia is a clinical sign that underlying problems need to be identified and corrected. In the ACLS arena, this arrhythmia can be the result of both ischemic and nonischemic events.

Thus, in the setting of fear, chest pain, and anxiety typical of AMI, the following actions are indicated:

- Oxygen administration
- IV access
- 12-lead ECG
- Pain relief with morphine and nitroglycerin

In contrast, volume and oxygenation problems are among the most common *nonischemic events* the ACLS provider will deal with. These patients often present with sinus tachycardia. For these patients, attention should be directed at the following fundamentals while other possible causes are searched for:

- 250 mL NS infusion
- Oxygen administration
- Intubation and ventilation as indicated

ACLS Intervention Sequence

As a healthy compensatory response, sinus tachycardia does not represent a treatable rhythm. Rather, it is a red flag warning of the existence of underlying problems.

In the setting of ACLS, sinus tachycardia may be an indication for one or more of the following nonspecific interventions:

- **Oxygen administration.** Oxygen is indicated for all patients with suspected AMI in the presence and the absence of respiratory distress.
- **Pain relief.** Morphine and nitroglycerin work synergistically on both anginal pain and its adverse hemodynamic effects.
- **Volume expansion.** Volume expansion is not part of the routine management of AMI. However, should evidence of volume depletion exist, a fluid challenge is indicated for its diagnostic and therapeutic benefits.
- **Intubation and ventilation.** Hypoxemia and hypoventilation are common causes of sinus tachycardia treatable with intubation, and hyperventilation with 100% oxygen.

ATRIAL FLUTTER

ECG Appearance

As illustrated in Figure 12–4, atrial flutter is the result of atrial ectopy *and* a re-entry loop that does *not* involve the AV node. The atria can be discharged 220 to 350 times per minute. It is remarkable, however, how often the atrial rate is right around 300/min.

Were all these impulses conducted to the ventricles, atrial flutter would be a lethal arrhythmia. Fortunately, the AV node with its built-in delay acts to block enough of these atrial ectopic P waves to prevent this from occurring.

It is common for patients with this arrhythmia to present to the emergency department with an atrial rate of about 300/min and a ventricular

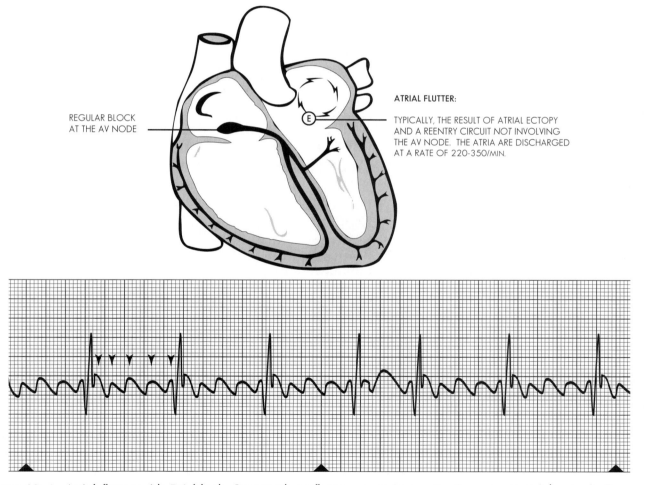

REGULAR BLOCK
AT THE AV NODE

ATRIAL FLUTTER:

TYPICALLY, THE RESULT OF ATRIAL ECTOPY
AND A REENTRY CIRCUIT *NOT* INVOLVING
THE AV NODE. THE ATRIA ARE DISCHARGED
AT A RATE OF 220-350/MIN.

Figure 12–4. Atrial flutter with 5:1 block. Saw tooth or flutter waves (see arrows) represent atrial ectopic P waves. Every fifth F wave is conducted except between the fourth and fifth R waves, where the conduction ratio is 3:1.

rate of 150/min. This is called atrial flutter with 2:1 AV conduction. The term 2:1 means that there are two ectopic P waves for each QRS. An example of this is seen in Figure 12–5.

Drugs with negative dromotropic effects act to slow conduction through the AV node. Thus, agents such as the beta blockers and the calcium channel blockers are used to produce 3:1, 4:1, or even 5:1 conduction ratios. These higher levels of block provide needed rate control. Figure 12–6 contains examples of atrial flutter with various conduction ratios and ventricular rates.

It can be seen that the ectopic P waves in atrial flutter have a characteristic shape or morphology. Called "*Flutter waves*" or "*F waves,*" they are often described as resembling a sawtooth or the tops of a picket fence. They are most prominent in leads II, III, and AVF.

Significance in ACLS

In the context of ACLS, acute episodes of atrial flutter are often the result of AMI.

Unwanted actions of digoxin and quinidine must also be considered as causes, as well as thyrotoxicosis and pulmonary embolus.

Atrial flutter with rates greater than 150/min will often result in pulmonary congestion and/or peripheral hypoperfusion if not treated promptly.

ACLS Intervention Sequence for Stable Atrial Flutter

When atrial flutter is not associated with serious signs and symptoms, the goal is to pharmacologically produce a ventricular response of between 60

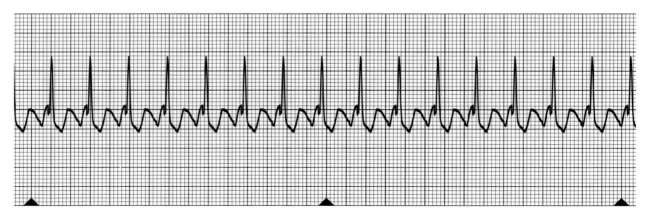

Figure 12–5. Atrial flutter with 2:1 AV conduction. The atrial rate is 300/min and the ventricular rate is 150/min. Thus, the AV node is successful in blocking half the ectopic atrial impulses. Without treatment, patients with ventricular rates higher than 150/min often develop CHF.

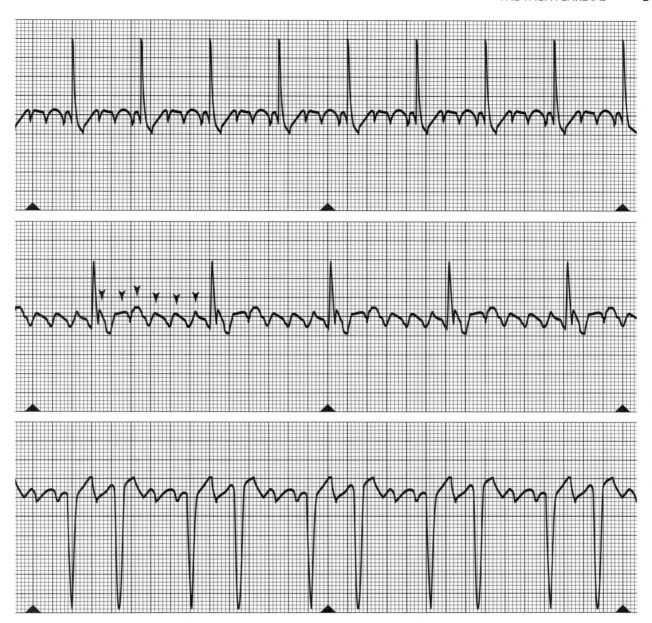

Figure 12–6. Examples of atrial flutter with various conduction ratios. It can be seen that as the conduction ratio goes up, the ventricular rate goes down. Since the atrial rate is usually right around 300, it can be noted that a 3:1 ratio will produce a ventricular rate of around 100/min. By the same token, a 4:1 ratio will often produce a rate of around 75/min. The 6:1 ratio in the middle example yields a rate of 50/min.

and 100 beats/min. The stable tachycardia algorithm recommends the following intervention sequence:

- Diltiazem for rate control
- Beta blockers for rate control
- Verapamil for rate control
- Digoxin for rate control
- Procainamide to prevent recurrence

- Quinidine to prevent recurrence
- Anticoagulants for chronic or unresponsive atrial flutter

ACLS Intervention Sequence for Unstable Atrial Flutter

If serious signs and symptoms are the result of atrial flutter, the ACLS provider must prepare for immediate synchronized cardioversion.

Recommendations for this procedure are presented in Figure 12–2, the electrical cardioversion algorithm. This pathway recommends the following energy sequence:

- 50 J
- 100 J
- 200 J
- 300 J
- 360 J

ATRIAL FIBRILLATION

ECG Appearance

Atrial fibrillation is the result of multiple ectopics and re-entry loops discharging the atria at rates of 350 to 600/min. Overwhelmed, the AV node loses its protective ability to block on a regular basis. The result is irregular depolarization of the ventricles.

Accordingly, atrial fibrillation has two electrocardiographic characteristics. These can be seen in Figure 12–7.

- **An irregular R–R interval.** Below the rhythm strip, the duration of each R–R interval is stated. You will note a wide variation in these intervals.
- **A fibrillatory line without discernible P waves.** Sometimes coarse, sometimes fine, but always fibrillatory, this line renders P waves unrecognizable.

Figure 12–8 demonstrates examples of atrial fibrillation with coarse and fine fibrillatory lines.

As with atrial flutter, congestive heart failure (CHF) is associated with ventricular rates greater than 150/min. In Figure 12–9, examples of atrial fibrillation with a rapid ventricular response are seen.

Significance in ACLS

In the context of ACLS, acute episodes of atrial fibrillation are often the result of AMI. Unwanted actions of digoxin and quinidine must also be con-

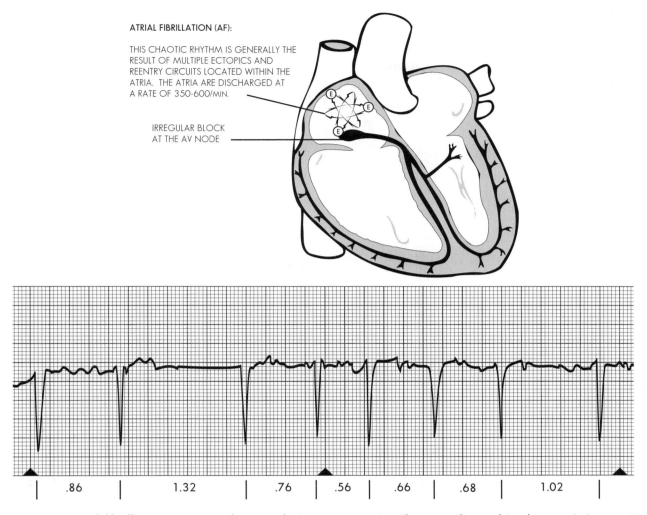

ATRIAL FIBRILLATION (AF):

THIS CHAOTIC RHYTHM IS GENERALLY THE RESULT OF MULTIPLE ECTOPICS AND REENTRY CIRCUITS LOCATED WITHIN THE ATRIA. THE ATRIA ARE DISCHARGED AT A RATE OF 350-600/MIN.

IRREGULAR BLOCK AT THE AV NODE

.86   1.32   .76   .56   .66   .68   1.02

Figure 12–7. Atrial fibrillation is an irregular irregularity. Its two major electrocardiographic characteristics are (1) an irregular R–R interval, and (2) a fibrillatory line without discernible P waves.

sidered, as well as less common causes such as thyrotoxicosis and pulmonary embolus.

Atrial fibrillation with rates greater than 150/min can result in pulmonary congestion and peripheral hypoperfusion if not treated promptly.

ACLS Intervention Sequence for Stable Atrial Fibrillation

When atrial fibrillation is not associated with serious signs and symptoms, the goal is to pharmacologically produce a ventricular response of between 60 and 100 beats/min. The stable tachycardia algorithm recommends the following intervention sequence:

- Diltiazem for rate control
- Beta blockers for rate control

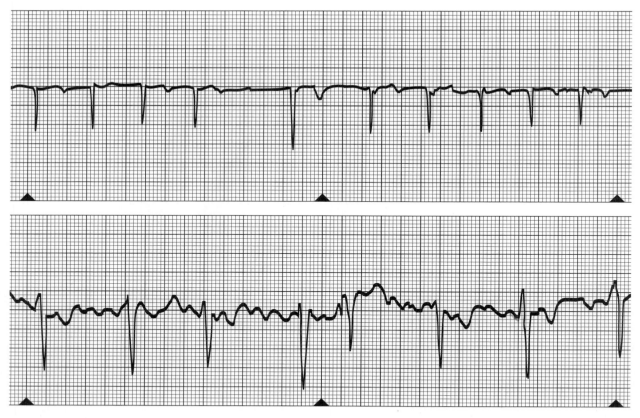

Figure 12–8. Examples of atrial fibrillation with coarse and fine fibrillatory lines.

- Verapamil for rate control
- Digoxin for rate control
- Procainamide to prevent recurrence
- Quinidine to prevent recurrence
- Anticoagulants for chronic or unresponsive atrial fibrillation

ACLS Intervention Sequence for Unstable Atrial Fibrillation

If serious signs and symptoms are the result of atrial fibrillation, the ACLS provider must prepare for immediate synchronized cardioversion.

The recommendations for this procedure are presented in Figure 12–2, the electrical cardioversion algorithm. This pathway presents the following energy sequence:

- 100 J
- 200 J
- 300 J
- 360 J

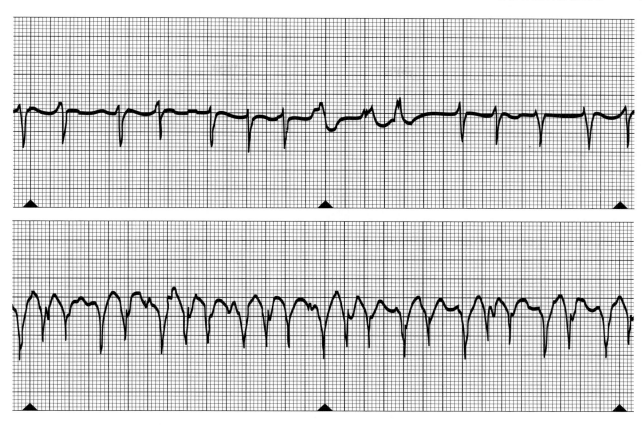

Figure 12–9. Examples of atrial fibrillation with a rapid ventricular response. It is hard to imagine either of these arrhythmias being associated with hemodynamic stability. The ventricular rate in the bottom example is 230/min. The broad complexes in the above examples represent aberrant conduction.

PAROXYSMAL SUPRAVENTRICULAR TACHYCARDIA (PSVT)

ECG Appearance

When three or more PACs occur in a row, atrial tachycardia is said to exist. As the term paroxysmal implies, PSVT is an arrhythmia that is distinguished from other forms of atrial tachycardia by its *sudden onset and recurrent nature.*

As depicted in Figure 12–10, episodes of PSVT are often triggered by a PAC that falls on or is *closely coupled* to the preceding T wave. Because it is generally the result of atrial ectopy and a re-entry circuit involving the AV node, *PSVT can often be terminated by vagal maneuvers.* Figure 12–11 shows an example of PSVT that was converted to a sinus rhythm by cartoid sinus massage.

The ECG characteristics of PSVT that can be noted in Figures 12–10 and 12–11 are as follows:

- The rate is typically between 140 and 220/min.
- The conduction ratio is 1:1. Thus, P waves are followed by QRS complexes.

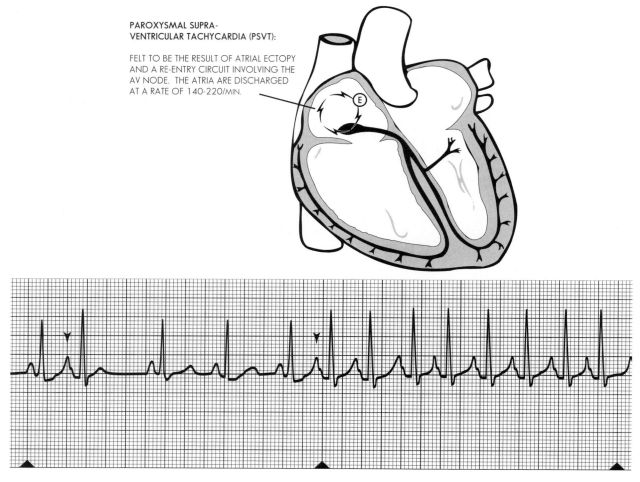

PAROXYSMAL SUPRA-
VENTRICULAR TACHYCARDIA (PSVT):

FELT TO BE THE RESULT OF ATRIAL ECTOPY
AND A RE-ENTRY CIRCUIT INVOLVING THE
AV NODE. THE ATRIA ARE DISCHARGED
AT A RATE OF 140-220/MIN.

Figure 12–10. Paroxysmal supraventricular tachycardia. The second PAC (see arrow) is closely coupled to the preceding T wave and triggers a run of PSVT. As its name implies, this arrhythmia is characterized by its precipitous onset.

- The rhythm is regular.
- The P waves are buried in the preceding T wave and are not usually visible.
- The QRS complexes are typically narrow. Occasionally bundle branch block or other aberrant conduction will exist and the rhythm will present with wide complexes. When this is the case, PSVT can be very difficult to differentiate from ventricular tachycardia.

Figure 12–12 displays various examples of PSVT. Note that this arrhythmia is a *regular irregularity with a normal QRS*.

Atrial Tachycardia with Block

There is a form of *nonparoxysmal* supraventricular tachycardia with which the ACLS provider should be familiar. Atrial tachycardia with 2:1 block is

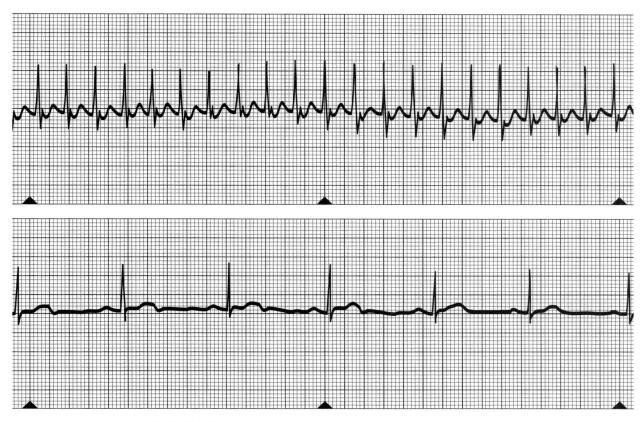

Figure 12–11. Conversion of PSVT following vagal stimulation. Cartoid sinus massage and facial ice water immersion may provide effective conversion of PSVT. In this example, PSVT with a rate of 180/min is converted to a sinus rhythm with a rate of 56/min.

common enough to deserve mention. Depicted in Figure 12–13, it is associated with digitalis intoxication. Like second-degree type II 2:1 AV block, there are two P waves for each QRS complex. However, there are two important differences:

- The atrial rate is 140 to 220/min. In second-degree type II 2:1 AV block, the atrial rate is sinus in origin and between 60 and 100/min.
- The QRS complex is normal. In second-degree type II block, the complexes are typically broad.

Significance of PSVT in ACLS

When this arrhythmia is the result of an acute ischemic event, the rapid heart rate often leads to serious signs and symptoms.

Chest pain, respiratory distress, and hypotension are indications that the patient should be prepared for immediate cardioversion.

A problem in ACLS is the differentiation between ventricular tachycardia and PSVT with aberrant conduction. This distinction is of more than

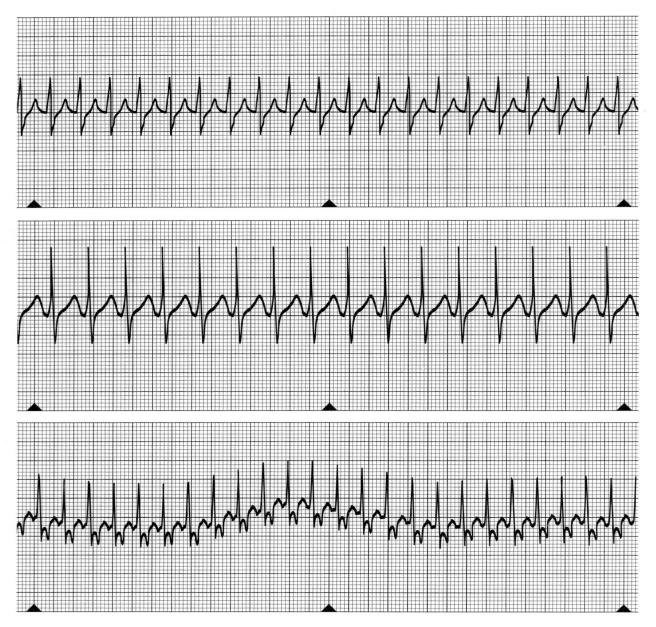

Figure 12–12. Examples of PSVT that meets stated standard criteria. Above are three examples of PSVT with rates of 155/min, 190/min, and 225/min, respectively. Note that the rhythm is regular, the QRS is normal, and P waves are not visible.

academic interest since administration of verapamil, or other calcium channel blocking agents, to a patient with VT can be a lethal error.

The tachycardia algorithms, however, provide two common sense guidelines to help prevent delays or mistakes in treatment:

- If serious signs and symptoms are present, the patient should be prepared for immediate cardioversion.
- If the complex appears to be wide, treat the rhythm like VT.

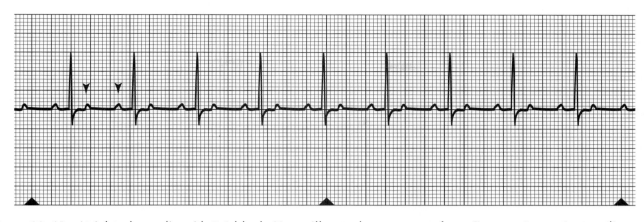

Figure 12–13. Atrial tachycardia with 2:1 block. You will note the presence of two P waves (arrows) preceding each normal QRS complex. In this arrhythmia, P waves occur 140 to 220 times/min. In 2:1 second-degree (type II) AV block, P waves are usually seen 60 to 100 times/min.

ACLS Intervention Sequence for Stable PSVT

If the patient does *not* display serious signs and symptoms, the guidelines recommend the following treatment sequence:

- Vagal maneuvers (Carotid sinus massage is contraindicated in patients with *carotid bruits*. Facial ice water immersion should be avoided in patients presenting with possible AMI.)
- Adenosine 6 mg rapid IV push.
- Adenosine 12 mg rapid IV push after 1 to 2 min (may repeat once after 1–2 min).
- Verapamil 2.5 to 5.0 mg IV *if complex is normal.*
- Lidocaine 1.0 to 1.5 mg IV *if complex is wide.*

ACLS Intervention Sequence for Unstable PSVT

If hemodynamic instability is the result of PSVT, the patient should be prepared for immediate cardioversion. The recommended energy sequence is:

- 50 J
- 100 J
- 200 J
- 300 J
- 360 J

PREMATURE VENTRICULAR CONTRACTIONS (PVCs)

Significance in ACLS

Despite the fact that PVCs are commonly seen following AMI, the JAMA guidelines do *not* support routine treatment of asymptomatic PVCs (Figure 12–14).

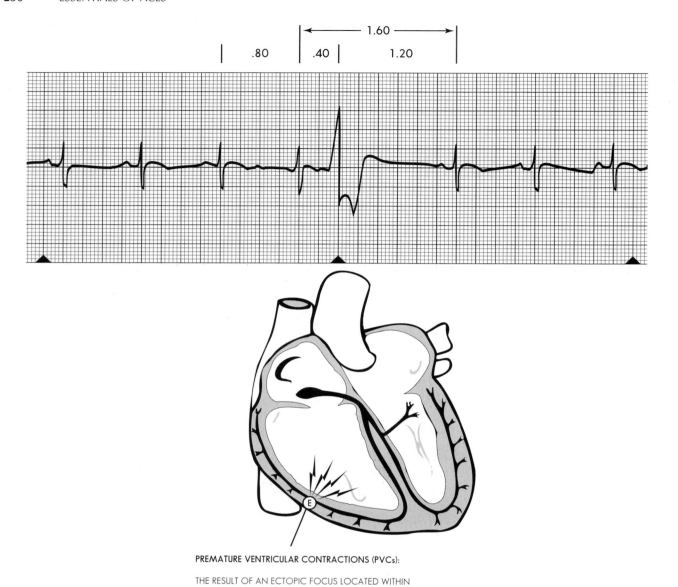

PREMATURE VENTRICULAR CONTRACTIONS (PVCs):

THE RESULT OF AN ECTOPIC FOCUS LOCATED WITHIN
THE VENTRICLES.

Figure 12–14. A single premature ventricular contraction. Note the typical complete compensatory pause. In the setting of possible AMI, the JAMA guidelines do not recommend routine treatment of symptomatic PVCs.

Once thought to forewarn VF or VT, their presence is now believed to indicate the need to deal with underlying problems.

Acute myocardial ischemia and injury are problems that require treatment with oxygen, morphine, nitroglycerin, aspirin, and thrombolytic agents.

In this context, ventricular ectopy can be both precipitated and amplified by electrolyte disturbances. Rapid identification and treatment of hypomagnesemia and hypokalemia is thus an important part of this picture.

Lidocaine and procainamide, by raising the fibrillatory threshold, will usually suppress ventricular ectopy in these patients. The danger is that by masking an important symptom, the ACLS provider can be lulled into a false sense of security.

Of course, at some point PVCs are symptomatic. A clinical marker no longer, they become a part of the problem and as such require antiarrhythmic therapy.

The guidelines state that patients who are myocardially infarcting *and* who display fresh onset *symptomatic* ventricular ectopy are appropriate candidates for antiarrhythmic therapy.

ECG Appearance

PVCs are the result of one or more ectopic foci located in the ventricles. There are special terms used to describe the electrocardiographic appearance of PVCs. They include:

- Infrequent (< 6/min)
- Frequent (> 6/min)
- Multifocal
- Couplets or pairs
- Bi- and trigeminal (so named when every second or third beat is a PVC)
- Salvos of VT (ventricular tachycardia is defined as three or more PVCs in a row)

Below in Figures 12–15 through 12–20 are examples of each of these types.

ACLS Intervention Sequence for Symptomatic PVCs

In the setting of possible AMI, PVCs should first be treated by therapeutic modalities aimed at reducing ischemia or by correcting established electrolyte abnormalities. This list includes:

- Oxygen
- Morphine

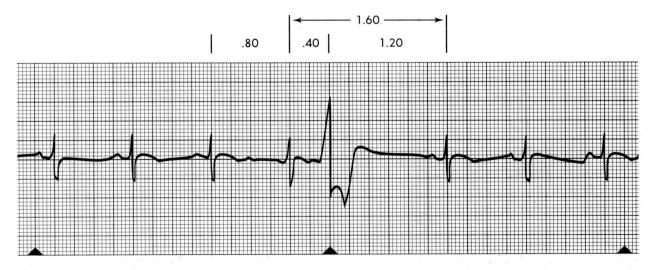

Figure 12–15. Infrequent PVCs.

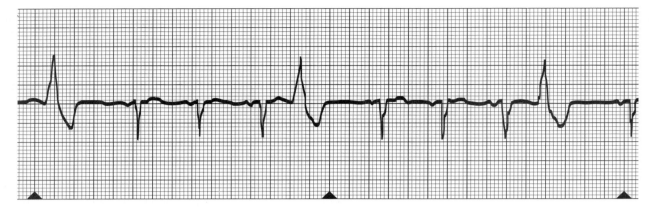

Figure 12–16. Frequent PVCs (> 6/min).

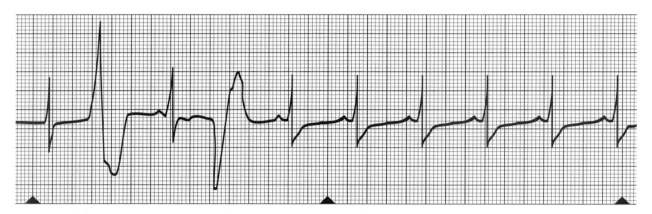

Figure 12–17. Multifocal PVCs.

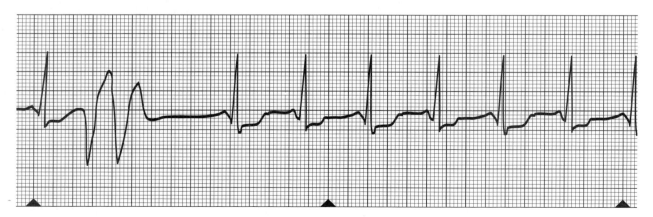

Figure 12–18. Coupled or paired PVCs.

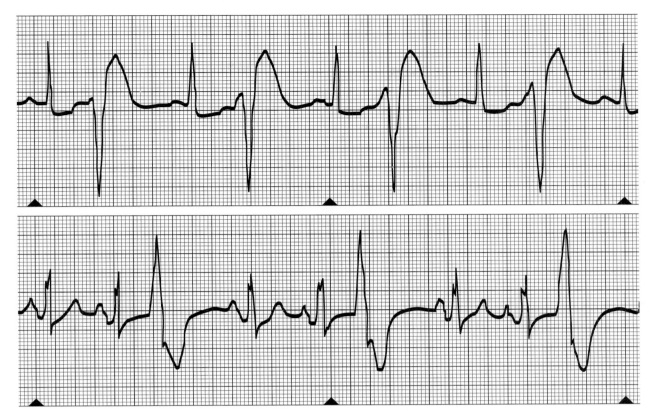

Figure 12–19. Bi- and trigeminal PVCs.

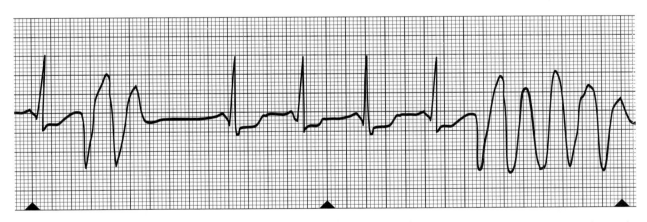

Figure 12–20. Salvos of ventricular tachycardia. Three or more PVCs occurring in a row define ventricular tachycardia (VT). Short runs are called bursts or salvos. Runs lasting more than 30 seconds are called sustained VT.

- Nitroglycerin
- Beta blockers
- Aspirin
- Thrombolytics
- Magnesium sulfate
- Potassium chloride

For patients not responding to the above therapy or whose symptoms are believed to be related to ventricular ectopy, the following antiarrhythmic sequence is recommended:

- Lidocaine 1.0 to 1.5 mg/kg IV push.
- Additional lidocaine boluses of 0.5 to 1.5 mg/kg every 5 to 10 min up to a maximum dose of 3.0 mg/kg.
- Lidocaine continuous infusion at 2 to 4 mg/kg.

VENTRICULAR TACHYCARDIA (VT)

ECG Appearance

Ventricular tachycardia is defined as three or more PVCs in a row. It is the result of one or more ventricular ectopic foci firing at a rate of 100 to 220/min.

This rhythm is generally regular in appearance. P waves may be present but are usually obscured by the rapid and broad ventricular complexes.

Short runs of VT are often called bursts or salvos. Runs that last more than 30 seconds can be called sustained VT (Figure 12–21). Runs that do not respond to therapeutic intervention are termed refractory.

Figure 12–22 displays examples of VT. Please note its characteristic appearance.

Ventricular tachycardia, like ventricular fibrillation, may by triggered by a PVC that lands on the T wave of the preceding complex. Figure 12–23 depicts an example of the R-on-T phenomenon.

Torsade de Pointes/Polymorphic VT

Torsade de pointes means *twisting of the points*. The term describes the appearance of this form of polymorphic VT. As can be seen from Figure 12–24, this arrhythmia waxes and wanes in amplitude and may "flip" or "twist" on its electrical axis.

Torsade de pointes is often caused by intoxication with drugs that prolong repolarization. These include the type 1A antiarrhythmics *procainamide, quinidine*, and *disopyramide*. Other agents with this side effect include the *tricyclic antidepressants* and the *phenothiazines*. This arrhythmia can also be caused by hypomagnesemia. Treatment is different from other forms of VT and consists of the following interventions:

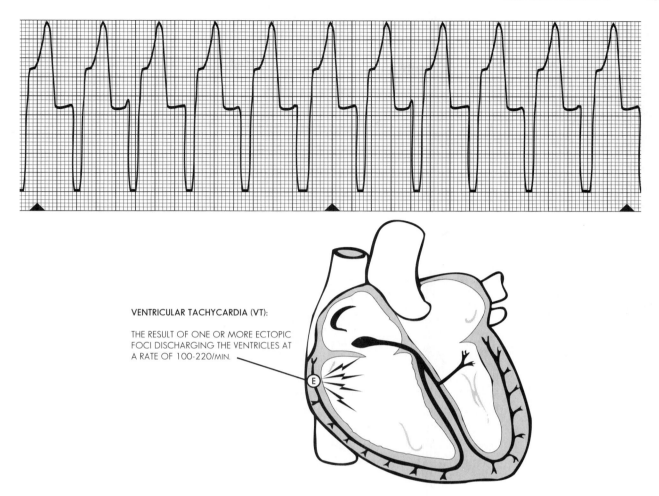

VENTRICULAR TACHYCARDIA (VT):

THE RESULT OF ONE OR MORE ECTOPIC FOCI DISCHARGING THE VENTRICLES AT A RATE OF 100-220/MIN.

Figure 12–21. Ventricular tachycardia is defined as three or more PVCs in a row occurring at a rate of 100 to 220/min. Runs lasting more than 30 seconds are called sustained VT.

- **If patient stability and time permit:**
  1 to 2 g magnesium sulfate over 1 to 2 minutes
  Overdrive pacing is also an acceptable option.
- **If unstable or pulseless Torsade de pointes is present:**
  Treat like VF (defibrillate at 200 J, 200 to 300 J, 360 J)

Significance of VT in ACLS

If not treated promptly, patients with VT rapidly develop CHF and systemic arterial hypotension. Cardiac arrest can develop if unstable VT is not treated promptly. Pulseless VT must be treated like VF.

ACLS Intervention Sequence for Stable VT

If the patient is clinically stable and not hypotensive, pharmacologic therapy should be initiated according to the stable tachycardia algorithm (Figure 12–1):

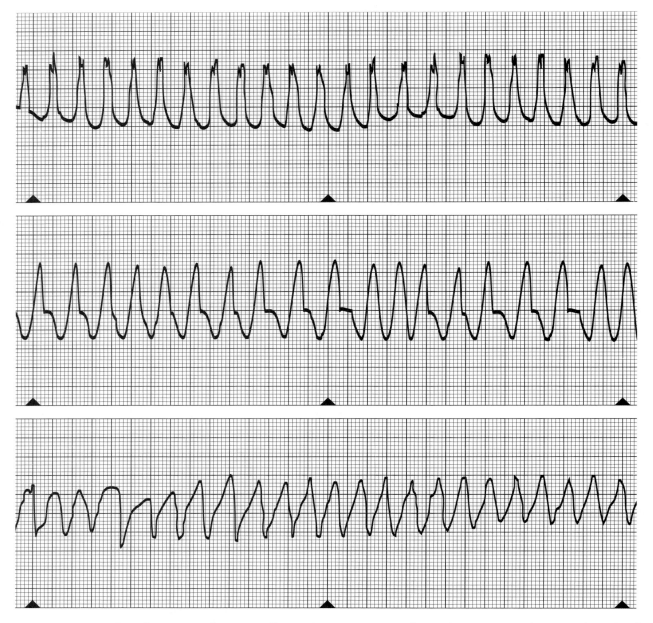

Figure 12–22. Examples of VT. Note the generally regular appearance of VT. The QRS complexes are broad reflecting its ventricular ectopic origin.

- Lidocaine 1.0 to 1.5 mg/kg IV push every 5 to 10 min.
- Lidocaine 0.5 to 0.75 mg/kg IV push (maximum dose 3 mg/kg).
- Procainamide 20 to 30 mg/min (maximum dose 17 mg/kg).
- Bretylium 5 to 10 mg/kg over 8 to 10 min (maximum dose 30 mg/kg over 24 hours).

ACLS Intervention Sequence for Unstable VT

If the patient is hypotensive or is experiencing other serious signs and symptoms of pump failure, preparation should be made for immediate syn-

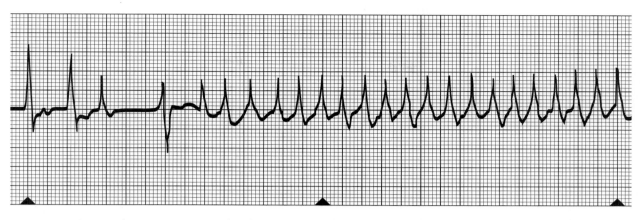

Figure 12–23. Onset of VT. Here a PVC lands on the T wave of the preceding supraventricular complex. The next complex shows aberrant conduction and another PVC lands on its T wave. This results in the abrupt onset of VT at a rate of approximately 240/min.

chronized cardioversion. The energy sequence recommended in Figure 12–2, the electrical cardioversion algorithm:

- 100 J
- 200 J
- 300 J
- 360 J

The guidelines emphasize that if delays in synchronization occur and clinical conditions are critical, the ACLS provider should immediately go to unsynchronized shocks.

ACLS Intervention for Pulseless VT

Pulseless VT must be treated like VF. Therefore, the synchronizer switch must be turned off and defibrillation performed immediately. The sequence is:

- 200 J
- 200 to 300 J
- 360 J
- Epinephrine/shock
- Lidocaine/shock
- Bretylium/shock
- Procainamide/shock
- Magnesium sulfate/shock

WIDE-COMPLEX TACHYCARDIAS OF UNCERTAIN ORIGIN

Figure 12–1, the stable tachycardia algorithm, contains a column with the heading *wide-complex tachycardia of uncertain type*. A nondistinct electro-

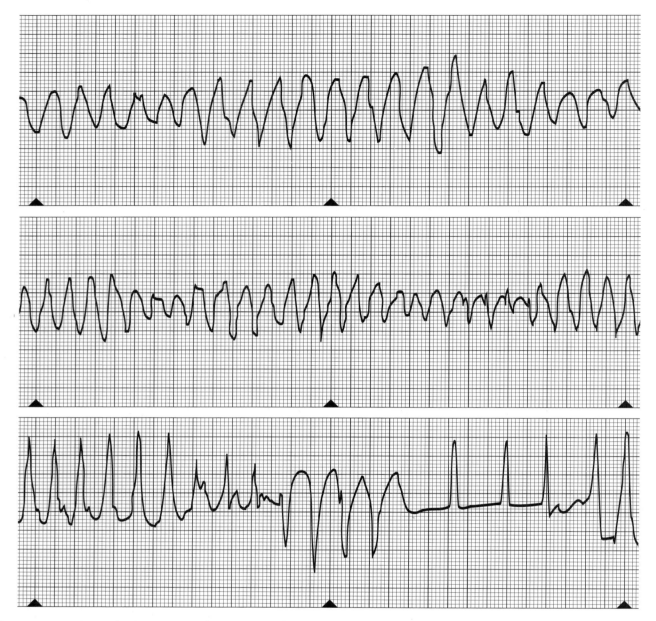

Figure 12–24. Torsade de pointes. This surprisingly common form of VF is characterized by waxing and waning of complex amplitude and by twisting of the electrical axis. Caused by hypomagnesemia or by antiarrhythmic drugs that prolong depolarization and the QT interval, this arrhythmia is treated with magnesium sulfate and/or overdrive pacing if patient stability and time permit. If serious signs and symptoms exist, this rhythm should be treated like VF.

cardiographic entity somewhere between PSVT and VT, these arrhythmias can present considerable confusion to the ACLS provider. A glance at the ECGs in Figure 12–25 confirms this statement.

Without sophisticated electrophysiologic tests not available in the ACLS setting, it may be impossible to distinguish PSVT with aberrant conduction from VT. This differentiation can be vitally important because the administration of verapamil to patients with VT can be a *lethal error.*

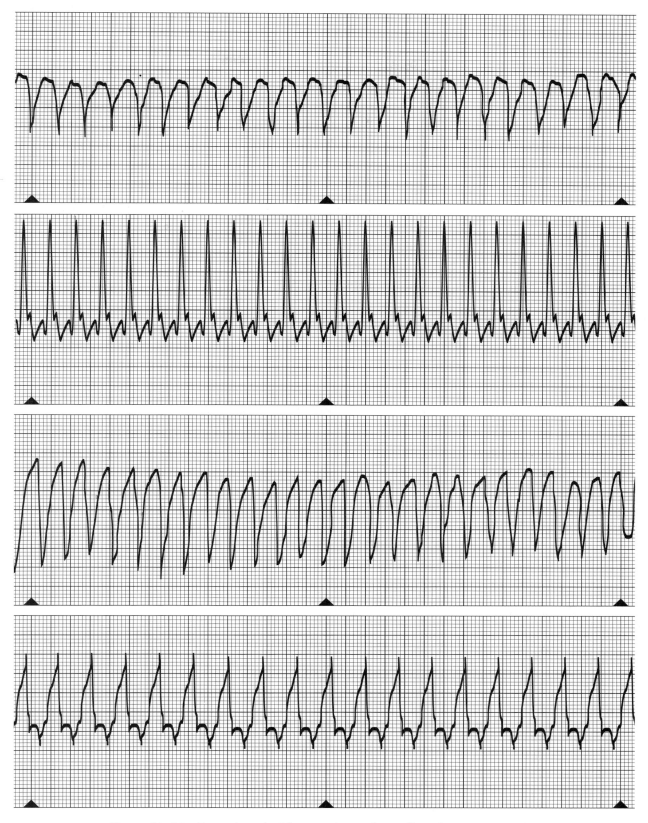

Figure 12–25. Examples of wide-complex tachycardias of uncertain origin.

Fortunately, the tachycardia algorithms are designed so that verapamil can *only* be administered to patients with narrow-complex tachycardias who are *not* hypotensive. Together, the tachycardia algorithms force the ACLS provider to come to two conclusions. Not surprisingly, these points direct the clinician away from the monitor and focus attention on the patient. These "rules" for managing tachycardias are as follows:

- **Rule 1.** If the patient is unstable as determined by the presence of serious signs and symptoms, *preparations must be made for immediate cardioversion.*
- **Rule 2.** If the QRS complex does not appear to be narrow, *treat the rhythm like VT.*

Further basing this approach in common sense, the JAMA guidelines stress that over 80% of wide complex tachycardias are due to VT.

Wide-complex Tachycardias Other Than PSVT or VT

Tachycardias other than PSVT and VT may present with wide complexes due to bundle branch block or other aberrant conduction. Figure 12–26 depicts sinus tachycardia with a wide complex. In this example, the P wave is not readily apparent.

Because lidocaine and cardioversion are not part of the treatment of sinus tachycardia, failure to closely inspect this rhythm could lead to harm.

Figure 12–27 shows an example of atrial fibrillation with a rapid ventricular response. Because the complex appears wide, this rhythm might mistakenly be treated with lidocaine according to the wide complex of uncertain origin intervention sequence.

This is where your calipers will prove indispensible! Remember, PSVT and VT are *regular irregularities.* In their case, the R–R interval is essentially unchanged from beat to beat.

In contrast, atrial fibrillation is *defined* by the presence of an irregular

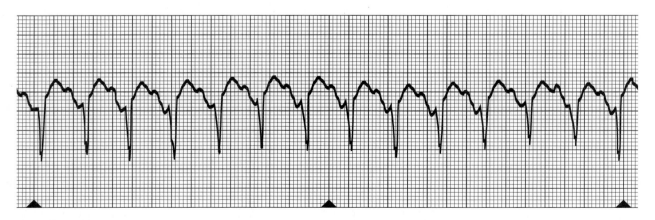

Figure 12–26. Wide-complex sinus tachycardia. Failure to inspect this ECG closely could lead to harm because electrical and pharmacologic therapy are not indicated. Sinus tachycardia is a healthy compensatory response which is usually rendered unnecessary by administration of oxygen, treatment of myocardial ischemia, and volume infusion if indicated.

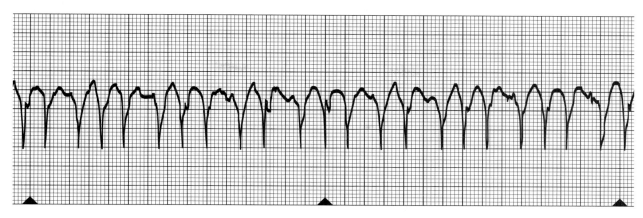

Figure 12–27. Wide-complex atrial fibrillation with a rapid ventricular response. Get out your calipers! The irregularity of the R–R interval defines this ECG as atrial fibrillation, not PSVT or VT.

R–R interval. Once again, careful inspection and thoughtful interpretation can assure proper therapy is given.

The JAMA guidelines state that faced with urgent care of an ill patient, the physician should ignore detailed criteria for ECG analysis and attend to the patient. This is not to say, as the two previous examples show, that careful analysis of the ECG is not of value. It *is* to say that the ACLS provider is charged with making the critical distinction between academic questions and clinical necessities.

ACLS Intervention Sequence for Stable Wide-complex Tachycardias of Uncertain Origin

Figure 12–1, the tachycardia algorithm, recommends the following sequence for these arrhythmias. You will notice the absence of verapamil.

- Lidocaine 1.0 to 1.5 mg/kg IV push every 5 to 10 min.
- Lidocaine 0.5 to 0.75 mg/kg IV push (maximum dose 3 mg/kg).
- Adenosine 6 mg rapid IV push over 1 to 3 sec.
- Adenosine 12 mg rapid IV push over 1 to 3 sec (may repeat once in 1 to 2 min).
- Procainamide 20 to 30 mg/min (maximum dose 17 mg/kg).
- Bretylium 5 to 10 mg/kg over 8 to 10 min (maximum dose 30 mg/kg over 24 hours).

BIBLIOGRAPHY

1. American Heart Association, Emergency Cardiac Care Committee and Subcommittees. Guidelines for cardiopulmonary resuscitation and emergency cardiac care. JAMA 1992;268:2171–2295
2. American Heart Association. Textbook of advanced cardiac life support. Dallas, TX: American Heart Association, 1994
3. American Heart Association. Instructor's manual for advanced cardiac life support. Dallas, TX: American Heart Association, 1994

4. Brugada P, Brugada J, Mont L, et al. A new approach to the differential diagnosis of regular tachycardia with wide QRS complex. Circulation 1991;83: 1649–1659

5. Herbert ME, Votey SR, Morgan MT, Cameron P, Dziukas L. Failure to agree on the electrocardiographic diagnosis of ventricular tachycardia. Ann Emerg Med 1996;27:35–38

6. Lowenstein SR, Halperin BD, Reiter MJ, et al: Paroxysmal supraventricular tachycardias. Journal of Emergency Medicine 1996;14:39–51

7. Pritchett EL, Management of atrial fibrillation. N Engl J Med 1992;326:1264–1271

8. Steinman RT, Herrera C, Schuger CD, et al. Wide QRS tachycardia in the conscious adult: ventricular tachycardia is the most frequent cause. JAMA 1989; 261:1013–1016

9. Steurer G, Gursot S, Frey B, et al: The differential diagnosis on the electrocardiogram between ventricular tachycardia and preexcited tachycardia. Clin Card 1994;17:306

10. Wrenn K. Management strategies in wide QRS complex tachycardia. Am J Emerg Med 1991;9:592–597

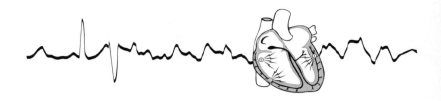

13. The Essential ACLS Cases

OVERVIEW

As discussed in Chapter 1, ACLS Course Requirements, completion of a "basic" ACLS course requires participants to successfully manage each of the nine essential ACLS cases. The guidelines and performance requirements for each of these cases are set forth in the American Heart Association's *Instructor's Manual for Advanced Cardiac Life Support*.

The blueprints for these cases are the nine core ACLS algorithms. Because their recommendations encourage appropriate flexibility, each patient care scenario can be tailored to suit course participants' educational needs.

Rounding out this review of adult ACLS, Chapter 13 summarizes the specifications for each required ACLS case. Accordingly, specific proficiency requirements for each are presented in the following format.

- The Case Setting
- The Case Scenario

- What you MUST do
- What you must NOT do

CASE 1: RESPIRATORY ARREST WITH A PULSE/THE UNIVERSAL ALGORITHM

Case Setting

Guidelines set forth in the American Heart Association's *Instructor's Manual for Advanced Cardiac Life Support*, recommend that Case 1: Respiratory Arrest With a Pulse, be placed in one or more of the following settings:

- An unmonitored pre-hospital setting
- An unmonitored emergency department setting
- An unmonitored hospital setting
- A monitored critical care unit setting

Therein, a variety of patient care scenarios can be presented to evaluate the *IV access* and *airway management skills* necessary to manage the unresponsive patient who is in respiratory, but *not* cardiac, arrest.

The Scenario

This case is designed to evaluate course participants' understanding of Figure 13–1, the universal algorithm. This case focuses on the airway management, assessment, and IV access skills necessary to manage unresponsive patients who are in respiratory, but *not* cardiac, arrest.

Course participants will be asked to demonstrate proper usage of all core noninvasive and invasive airway management techniques as described in Chapter 3. Participants will also be asked to demonstrate IV access techniques as described in Chapter 5.

Critical Performance Skills

What You MUST Do

In order to demonstrate proficiency at this station the following critical actions as outlined in the universal algorithm must be performed:

- Perform initial assessment using the steps of the primary ABCD survey depicted in the universal algorithm:
    Determine unresponsiveness/call for help
    Open the airway
    Look, listen, and feel for breathing
    Give two slow breaths
    Determine presence of pulse
    Perform rescue breathing
- Demonstrate the ability to properly utilize the following *noninvasive* airway management techniques and equipment:
    Jaw thrust and alternative airway opening technique
    Barrier devices

Universal Algorithm for Adult
Emergency Cardiac Care

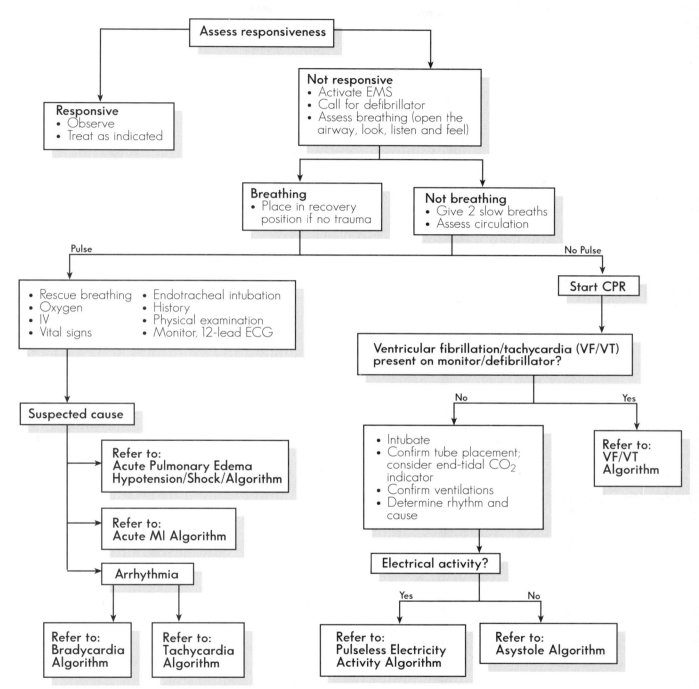

Figure 13–1. The universal algorithm. The critical actions for Case 1: Respiratory Arrest With a Pulse, are detailed in this algorithm. (Algorithm copyright 1992, American Medical Association; JAMA, October 28, 1992; pp 2199–2241.)

Oropharyngeal and nasopharangeal airways
Bag–valve–mask ventilation
Simple oxygen masks
Non-rebreathing mask
Nasal cannula
Face mask ventilation with and without supplemental oxygen
Suctioning techniques

- Demonstrate the ability to properly perform endotracheal intubation
- Demonstrate the following with regard to endotracheal intubation:
  Ability to properly assess endotracheal tube placement by use of auscultation and end-tidal CO_2 devices
  Knowledge of the hazards and complications of the procedure
- Demonstrate the following with regard to providing IV access:
  Advantages of peripheral access
  Selection of site
  Proper IV access techniques
  Choice of proper IV fluid
- Demonstrate an understanding of the need to assess the patient requiring ACLS as regards:
  The "ABC's"
  Proper functioning of oxygen and IV devices
  Cardiac monitoring
  Vital signs
  History and physical
  12-lead ECG
  Laboratory determinations
- Demonstrate the ability to arrange for postresuscitation care to include *continuous ventilatory support*

What You Must NOT Do

The AHA's *Instructor's Manual for ACLS* cites the following actions as unacceptable performance errors:

- Failure to determine the presence of respiratory arrest without cardiac arrest
- Initiating compressions, drugs, or defibrillation in this scenario
- Performing rescue breathing inappropriately
- Failure to properly provide oxygen, cardiac monitoring, and IV access in this scenario
- Performing endotracheal intubation in an unsafe manner
  Not hyperventilating and hyperoxygenating prior to attempts
  Attempts that last more than 30 seconds
- Failure to recognize endobronchial or esophageal intubation
- Failure to recognize the need for continuous assessment of this and *all* patients requiring ACLS to include:

ABCs
Vital signs
History and physical
12-lead ECG
Laboratory data

CASE 2: WITNESSED CARDIAC ARREST/THE AED ALGORITHM

Case Setting

Guidelines set forth in the American Heart Association's *Instructor's Manual for Advanced Cardiac Life Support* recommend that Case 2: Witnessed Cardiac Arrest/AED Management, be placed in one or more of the following settings:

- An unmonitored pre-hospital setting
- An unmonitored emergency department setting
- An unmonitored hospital setting
- A monitored critical care unit setting

Therein, a variety of patient care scenarios can be presented to evaluate course participants' ability to manage a witnessed adult cardiac arrest using an automated external defibrillator (AED).

The Scenario

This case is designed to evaluate understanding of the management of adult cardiac arrest using automated external defibrillator devices (AEDs).

These principles are highlighted in Figure 13–2, the AED critical pathway. This intervention sequence focuses on the victim who requires multiple sets of shocks from an AED device.

According to the ACLS instructor's manual, Case 2 is designed to emphasize a fundamental ACLS concept: *The passage of time drives all aspects of ECG!* Therefore, to successfully manage this "patient," CPR and defibrillation must be performed *within 90 seconds* of collapse.

If this critical performance skill is accomplished, the hypothetical patient will convert to a perfusing rhythm with a palpable pulse and adequate blood pressure.

If defibrillation is *not* employed within 90 seconds, the "patient" will develop terminal asystole.

This case is designed to evaluate BLS and AED management skills only. ACLS interventions such as IV access, endotracheal intubation, and pharmacologic therapy are assessed in other cases.

Critical Performance Skills

What You MUST Do

In order to demonstrate proficiency at this station, the following critical actions must be performed:

Automated External Defibrillation (AED) Critical Pathway*

Step I: Verify need for defibrillation

- Determine presence of cardiac arrest
- Initiate CPR
- Attach AED
- Activate "analysis" control

Step II: Defibrillate three times if commanded
(200 J, 200-300 J, 360 J)

- Clear the patient
- Activate "analysis" after each shock
- Shock if commanded
- Check pulse if "no shock indicated" is displayed

Step III: Check pulse and perform CPR for 1 min.

- After one minute of CPR activate "analysis"

Step IV: Repeat three stacked shocks if commanded
(200 J, 200-300 J, 360 J)

- Clear the patient
- Activate "analysis" after each shock
- Shock if commanded
- Check pulse if "no shock indicated" is displayed

Step V: Check pulse and perform CPR for 1 min.

- After one minute of CPR activate "analysis"

Step VI: Repeat sets of three shocks and CPR as indicated

- Shock three times if commanded
- Check pulse and perform CPR for one minute if indicated
- Repeat as needed until the patient is no longer in cardiac arrest or VF is not detected

---

Figure 13–2. The AED critical pathway. Understanding of this critical pathway is evaluated in Case 2, Witnessed Adult Cardiac Arrest. *Please refer to the AED treatment algorithm in your AHA textbook of ACLD for additional information. (Algorithm copyright 1992, American Medical Association; JAMA, October 28, 1992; pp 2199–2241.)

- Perform initial assessment using the steps of the primary ABCD survey as depicted in the universal algorithm:
  Assess unresponsiveness/call for help
  Call for defibrillator
  Open airway/assess breathing/give two slow breaths
  Establish pulselessness
  Initiate CPR
- Properly attach and safely operate AED device. *Note:* The first shock must be delivered within 90 seconds!
  Properly place defibrillator pads in the *sternal–apex* positions
  Activate "power on" control
  Activate "analysis" control
  Do NOT perform CPR during analysis
  If shockable rhythm detected, *clear the patient!*
  Give set of three shocks if indicated pressing "analysis" after each shock
  Check pulse if "no shockable rhythm" message is displayed *or* after the third shock
  Demonstrate proper airway management using noninvasive techniques
  Recognize need to *check pulse* if "no shockable rhythm" message is displayed *and* after third, sixth, and ninth shocks
- Assess blood pressure if pulse is present
- Demonstrate the ability to monitor and support the patient postresuscitation
  Maintain airway and ventilate
  Oxygen, IV, monitor
  Assess vital signs

What You Must NOT Do

The AHA's *Instructor's Manual for ACLS* cites the following actions as unacceptable:

- Failure to properly assess using primary ABCD survey
- Performing CPR during rhythm analysis
- Failure to "clear the patient" prior to defibrillation
- Failing to properly check for pulse:
  If "no shock indicated" message is displayed
  After each set of three shocks

CASE 3: MEGA VF: REFRACTORY VF–PULSELESS VT/THE VF–VT ALGORITHM

Case Setting

Guidelines set forth in the current American Heart Association's *Instructor's Manual for Advanced Cardiac Life Support* recommend that this case revolve around a victim whose cardiac arrest is witnessed.

ACLS instructors are given the flexibility to choose from one or more of the following settings, depending on course participant needs.

- An unmonitored pre-hospital setting
- An unmonitored emergency department setting
- An unmonitored hospital setting
- A monitored critical care unit setting

The Scenario

Based on the critical actions contained in the VF/VT algorithm (Figure 13–3), this case forms the "core" around which other ACLS cases are structured. As VF/VT is responsible for the overwhelming majority of cardiac arrests, the primary goal of ACLS is to ensure early defibrillation to these victims. ACLS Case 3 is designed to emphasize these most vital skills. Accordingly, in this code station, course participants will be asked to manage the first 10 minutes of a witnessed adult cardiac arrest due to VF/VT.

Critical Performance Skills

What You MUST Do

The AHA's *Instructor's Manual for ACLS* stipulates that this case involves a witnessed cardiac arrest that may or may not have been monitored. As the initial rescuer to arrive at the scene, to demonstrate proficiency, the course participant must successfully perform the following actions:

- Using the guidelines of the universal algorithm and the primary ABCD survey, determine unconsciousness and pulselessness.
- Properly perform one-person CPR.
- Using a monitor defibrillator (which is available) determine the presence of VF or pulseless VT.
- Assess the presence of refractory VF/VT by failure to respond to three "stacked" unsynchronized countershocks.
- Direct additional rescuers *who arrive at this point* in the following interventions:
    CPR
    Intubation
    Peripheral IV access
- Demonstrate effective team leadership by properly instructing the "code team" as to the proper utilization of endotracheal intubation in cardiac arrest:
    Proper technique
    Role in maintaining acid–base balance
    Role, dosages, etc. as drug administration route
- Demonstrate effective team leadership by properly directing the code team as to the proper dosage administration technique, intervention sequence, and hazards of the following agents:
    Epinephrine
    Lidocaine
    Bretylium

Ventricular Fibrillation/Pulseless Ventricular Tachycardia (VF/VT) Algorithm

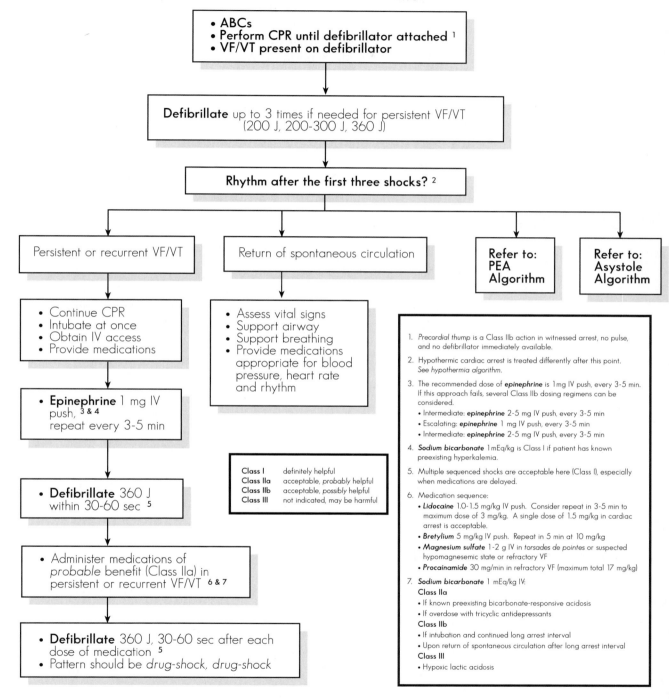

Figure 13–3. The VF/VT algorithm. The critical actions for Case 3, Mega VF: Refractory VF/VT, are detailed in this algorithm. (Algorithm copyright 1992, American Medical Association; JAMA, October 28, 1992; pp 2199–2241.)

Procainamide
Magnesium sulfate
Sodium bicarbonate
- Defibrillate at 360 J within 30 to 60 seconds after each drug using a "drug–shock, drug–shock" pattern.
- Direct the code team to perform CPR between defibrillatory efforts
- Direct the code team in proper postresuscitation care to include:
Stopping CPR once a pulse is present
Evaluating blood pressure and hemodynamic stability
Properly identifying and managing tachycardias and bradycardias that may develop during the postresuscitation phase
Continuing to assess the primary ABCD survey and appropriately resuming CPR as necessary

What You Must NOT Do

The AHA *Instructor's Manual for ACLS* lists the following performance errors as being unacceptable:

- Forgetting to perform CPR whenever pulselessness exists.
- Not providing effective ventilation with the proper airway adjunct.
- Not intubating the trachea after determining the presence of refractory VF/VT
- Failure to defibrillate properly including:
Wrong energy level
Failure to "clear" patient or "stack" shocks
Failure to shock within 30 to 60 seconds after each drug
- Critical pharmacologic errors such as:
Wrong drug or sequence
Wrong dose
Wrong maximum dose
Failure to recognize hazards

CASE 4: PULSELESS ELECTRICAL ACTIVITY/THE PEA ALGORITHM

Case Setting

Guidelines set forth in the American Heart Association's *Instructor's Manual for Advanced Cardiac Life Support* recommend that Case 4, Pulseless Electrical Activity, be placed in one or more of the following settings:

- An unmonitored pre-hospital setting
- An unmonitored emergency department setting
- An unmonitored hospital setting
- A monitored critical care unit setting

Therein, a variety of patient care scenarios can be presented to evaluate the differential diagnosis of PEA and to correspondingly determine acceptable therapeutic interventions.

The Scenario

This case is designed to evaluate course participants' understanding of the pulseless electrical activity algorithm (Figure 13–4). Pulseless electrical activity (PEA) is defined as pulselessness with a rhythm other than VF/VT or asystole.

Pulseless Electrical Activity (PEA) Algorithm
(Electromechanical Dissociation [EMD])

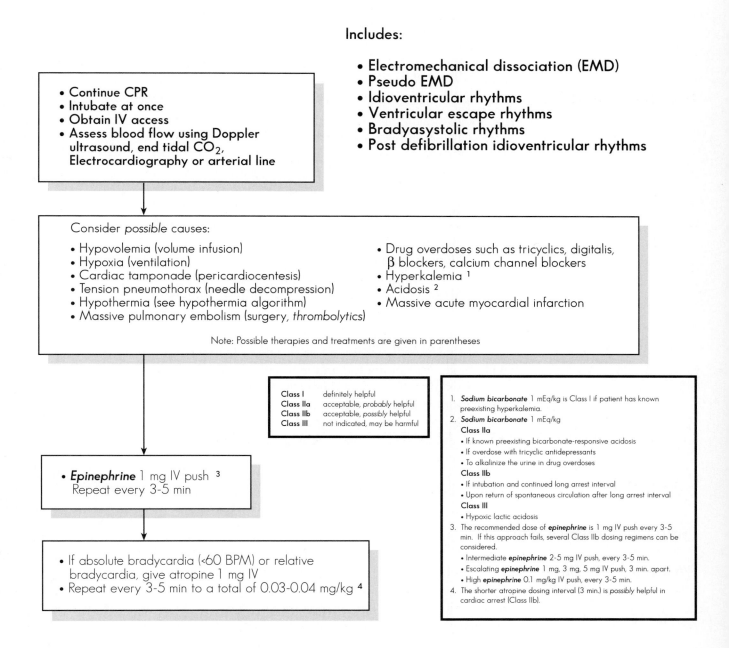

Includes:

- Electromechanical dissociation (EMD)
- Pseudo EMD
- Idioventricular rhythms
- Ventricular escape rhythms
- Bradyasystolic rhythms
- Post defibrillation idioventricular rhythms

- Continue CPR
- Intubate at once
- Obtain IV access
- Assess blood flow using Doppler ultrasound, end tidal CO_2, Electrocardiography or arterial line

Consider *possible* causes:

- Hypovolemia (volume infusion)
- Hypoxia (ventilation)
- Cardiac tamponade (pericardiocentesis)
- Tension pneumothorax (needle decompression)
- Hypothermia (see hypothermia algorithm)
- Massive pulmonary embolism (surgery, *thrombolytics*)

- Drug overdoses such as tricyclics, digitalis, β blockers, calcium channel blockers
- Hyperkalemia [1]
- Acidosis [2]
- Massive acute myocardial infarction

Note: Possible therapies and treatments are given in parentheses

Class I	definitely helpful
Class IIa	acceptable, *probably helpful*
Class IIb	acceptable, *possibly helpful*
Class III	not indicated, may be harmful

1. *Sodium bicarbonate* 1 mEq/kg is Class I if patient has known preexisting hyperkalemia.
2. *Sodium bicarbonate* 1 mEq/kg
   Class IIa
   - If known preexisting bicarbonate-responsive acidosis
   - If overdose with tricyclic antidepressants
   - To alkalinize the urine in drug overdoses
   Class IIb
   - If intubation and continued long arrest interval
   - Upon return of spontaneous circulation after long arrest interval
   Class III
   - Hypoxic lactic acidosis
3. The recommended dose of *epinephrine* is 1 mg IV push every 3-5 min. If this approach fails, several Class IIb dosing regimens can be considered.
   - Intermediate *epinephrine* 2-5 mg IV push, every 3-5 min.
   - Escalating *epinephrine* 1 mg, 3 mg, 5 mg IV push, 3 min. apart.
   - High *epinephrine* 0.1 mg/kg IV push, every 3-5 min.
4. The shorter atropine dosing interval (3 min.) is *possibly* helpful in cardiac arrest (Class IIb).

- *Epinephrine* 1 mg IV push [3]
  Repeat every 3-5 min

- If absolute bradycardia (<60 BPM) or relative bradycardia, give atropine 1 mg IV
- Repeat every 3-5 min to a total of 0.03-0.04 mg/kg [4]

Figure 13–4. The PEA algorithm. The critical actions for Case 4: Pulseless Electrical Activity, are detailed in this algorithm. (Algorithm copyright 1992, American Medical Association; JAMA, October 28, 1992; pp 2199–2241.)

As the PEA algorithm indicates, this problem is associated with a fairly large group of arrhythmias. Rhythms such as EMD and pseudo-EMD typically present with normal QRS complexes. Broad complex PEAs such as ventricular escape, idioventricular, bradyasystolic rhythms associated with unfavorable outcomes.

The major emphasis of this case is that PEA is caused by a wide variety of underlying entities, many of which can be treated successfully.

Thus, the main thing that must be done when confronted with PEA is to search for a treatable underlying cause.

Below, taken from the PEA algorithm, is a list of possible causes. You will note that next to them in parentheses is the designation "essential" or "comprehensive."

Typically, the differential diagnosis of the first four cases are emphasized in an essential ACLS course. Not coincidentally, these are the most common causes of PEA. The remaining causes and their management receive greater emphasis as part of a comprehensive ACLS course:

- Hypovolemia (essential)
- Hypoxia (essential)
- Cardiac tamponade (essential)
- Tension pneumothorax (essential)
- Hypothermia (comprehensive)
- Massive pulmonary embolism (comprehensive)
- Drug overdoses such as tricyclics, digitalis, beta blockers, calcium channel blockers (comprehensive)
- Hyperkalemia (comprehensive)
- Pre-existing acidosis (comprehensive)
- Massive acute myocardial infarction (comprehensive)

Hypovolemia is the most common cause of PEA. It is also easily treatable with a volume infusion.

Hypoxia is also a common problem. If this is the underlying cause, it will respond to intubation and ventilation with 100% oxygen.

Thus, the differential diagnosis of PEA includes a fluid challenge and ventilation with 100% oxygen.

This is a very wise approach because should these two common causes *not* be responsible, significant benefit will likely result from these interventions.

Thus, a fluid challenge along with CPR, intubation, and epinephrine administration, should be part of the routine management of PEA.

Critical Performance Skills

What You MUST Do

As described above, the most common causes of PEA are characteristically evaluated as part of an essential ACLS course. These four causes and their ACLS management are summarized below:

- Hypovolemia
    Treatment: Volume infusion
- Hypoxia (acute respiratory failure)
    Treatment: Intubation and ventilation
- Cardiac tamponade
    Treatment: Pericardiocentesis
- Tension pneumothorax
    Treatment: Needle decompression

However, regardless of underlying cause, the following *nonspecific* performance skills must be demonstrated:

- Determining the presence of PEA
- CPR
- Physical assessment to determine underlying cause
- Intubation and ventilation with 100% oxygen
- Providing IV access
- Volume infusion with 250 mL NS
- Use of epinephrine
- Use of atropine if the cardiac rate is less than 60/min

This performance station will present one or more scenarios to evaluate course participants' ability to initiate and conduct the differential diagnosis of PEA. Important features of these scenarios appear below:

Scenario 1: PEA Due to Hypovolemia

- Suggestive historical data
    Major abdominal or thoracic trauma
    Complaint of severe upper or lower GI fluid loss
    Macroscopic hematemesis or hematochezia
    Protracted poor nutritional status (IVDA or SNF admit)
    Obvious severe bleeding
    Diabetic crisis
    Overexposure or "heatstroke"

- Suggestive signs and symptoms
    Flat neck veins
    Properly performed CPR produces no or weak pulse
    Favorable response to volume infusion

- Therapeutic interventions
    Volume infusion/replacement
    Hemostasis
    Other targeted therapy where possible, eg, insulin

Scenario 2: PEA Due to Hypoxia and Acute Respiratory Failure

- Suggestive historical data
    History of COPD or other respiratory disease
    Recent difficult intubation
    Hypoxemia that does not respond to oxygen

- Suggestive signs and symptoms
    Abnormal breath sounds
    Apnea/tachycardia
    Cyanosis
    Severely decreased SaO_2
    Shortness of breath
- Therapeutic interventions
    Assure airway patency
    Intubation and ventilation with 100% oxygen
    Assure proper functioning of ventilator
    Assure proper placement of endotracheal tube

Scenario 3: PEA Due to Cardiac Tamponade

- Suggestive historical data
    Chest trauma, either penetrating or nonpenetrating
    Pulmonary infection
    Lung and/or breast cancer
    Recent CPR
    Recent chest pain
- Suggestive signs and symptoms
    Jugular venous distention (JVD)
    Properly performed CPR produces no or weak pulse
    Pericardial friction rub
    Pulsus paradoxus
    Echocardiogram if status permits
- Therapeutic interventions
    Volume infusion
    Pericardiocentesis

Scenario 4: PEA Due to Tension Pneumothorax

- Suggestive historical data
    Chest trauma
    Presence of central lines
    Receiving continuous ventilatory support
    Recent CPR
    Status asthmaticus or exacerbation of COPD
- Suggestive signs and symptoms
    Jugular venous distention (JVD)
    Tracheal deviation toward unaffected side
    Unilateral breath sounds
    No or weak pulse with properly performed CPR
    Respiratory distress
    Florid face
- Therapeutic interventions
    Needle decompression

What You Must NOT Do

The current *Instructor's Manual for ACLS* cites the following performance errors as unacceptable:

- Not assessing the patient
- Not performing an effective differential diagnosis process
- Treating only with epinephrine
- Not if bradycardia exists using atropine
- Not intubating and ventilating with 100% oxygen
- Not giving a volume infusion
- Defibrillating the patient with PEA
- Not performing CPR

CASE 5: ASYSTOLE/THE ASYSTOLE ALGORITHM

Case Setting

Guidelines set forth in the American Heart Association's *Instructor's Manual for ACLS* recommend that Case 5, Asystole, be placed in one or more of the following settings:

- An unmonitored pre-hospital setting
- An unmonitored emergency department setting
- An unmonitored hospital setting
- A monitored critical care unit setting

Therein, a variety of patient case scenarios can be presented to evaluate course participants' ability to perform the differential diagnosis of asystole and to correspondingly determine an acceptable therapeutic intervention sequence.

The Scenario

This case is based on the critical action outlined in Figure 13–5, the asystole algorithm. As emphasized in the current ACLS instructor's manual, this code station is designed to evaluate course participants' understanding of the following fundamental principals that guide the management of asystole:

1. Asystole usually represents a confirmation of death rather than a rhythm to be treated.
2. *Like* PEA, the ACLS provider must perform a differential diagnosis. *Unlike* PEA, treatable causes are relatively rare.
3. Intubation and ventilation along with CPR are the core interventions in maintaining acid–base balance in any cardiac arrest.
4. If ACLS providers are *unable* to find a treatable cause and if asystole does *not* respond to CPR intubation and drug therapy, the team leader must consider terminating code efforts.

Critical Performance Skills

What You MUST Do

Guidelines set forth in the AHA's *Instructor's Manual for ACLS* state that to demonstrate proficiency at this station, course participants must perform the following actions as outlined in Figure 13–5, the asystole algorithm:

- Assess cardiac arrest using primary ABCD survey skills
- Initiate and continue CPR
- Properly attach monitor/defibrillator
- Recognize asystole and *confirm its presence in more than one lead*
- Utilize *intubation* and *ventilation* with 100% oxygen as the primary means of achieving acid–base balance during CPR
- Obtain IV access
- Consider the following possible treatable causes of asystole, their differential diagnosis, and treatment where indicated:
    Hypoxia
    Hyperkalemia
    Hypokalemia
    Pre-existing acidosis
    Drug overdose
    Hypothermia
- Consider the immediate use of TCP and the guidelines for this intervention:
    It is *not* part of the routine treatment of asystole
    To be effective, it must be performed early and simultaneously with epinephrine and atropine
- Administer the following drugs as indicated, using proper dosage with awareness of limitations and hazards:
    Epinephrine
    Atropine
    Sodium bicarbonate
- Consider termination of code efforts if the following conditions exist:
    An underlying treatable cause is not found
    Asystole persists despite CPR, intubation, and proper medication sequencing

What You Must NOT Do

The AHA's *Instructor's Manual for ACLS* lists the following as unacceptable performance errors:

- Failure to confirm asystole in more than one lead
- Routine shocking of asystole
- Improper use of TCP
- Reliance on sodium bicarbonate to maintain acid–base balance

Asystole Treatment Algorithm

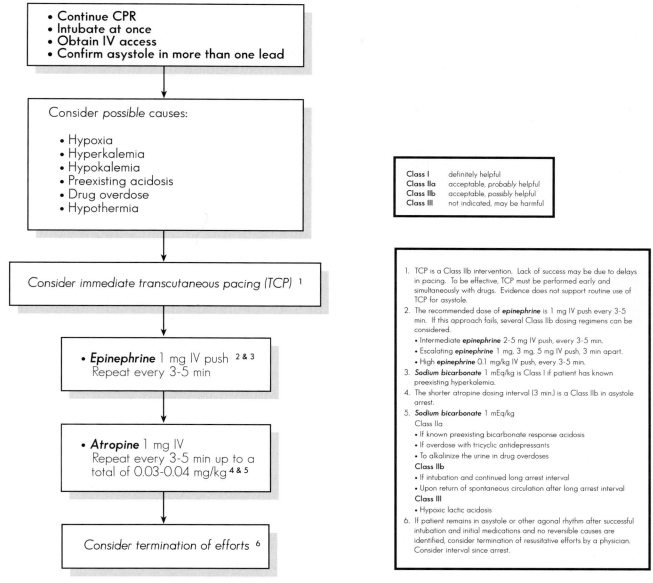

- Continue CPR
- Intubate at once
- Obtain IV access
- Confirm asystole in more than one lead

Consider *possible* causes:

- Hypoxia
- Hyperkalemia
- Hypokalemia
- Preexisting acidosis
- Drug overdose
- Hypothermia

Class I	definitely helpful
Class IIa	acceptable, *probably* helpful
Class IIb	acceptable, *possibly* helpful
Class III	not indicated, may be harmful

Consider immediate transcutaneous pacing (TCP) [1]

- *Epinephrine* 1 mg IV push [2 & 3]
  Repeat every 3-5 min

- *Atropine* 1 mg IV
  Repeat every 3-5 min up to a
  total of 0.03-0.04 mg/kg [4 & 5]

Consider termination of efforts [6]

1. TCP is a Class IIb intervention. Lack of success may be due to delays in pacing. To be effective, TCP must be performed early and simultaneously with drugs. Evidence does not support routine use of TCP for asystole.
2. The recommended dose of **epinephrine** is 1 mg IV push every 3-5 min. If this approach fails, several Class IIb dosing regimens can be considered.
   - Intermediate **epinephrine** 2-5 mg IV push, every 3-5 min.
   - Escalating **epinephrine** 1 mg, 3 mg, 5 mg IV push, 3 min apart.
   - High **epinephrine** 0.1 mg/kg IV push, every 3-5 min.
3. **Sodium bicarbonate** 1 mEq/kg is Class I if patient has known preexisting hyperkalemia.
4. The shorter atropine dosing interval (3 min.) is a Class IIb in asystole arrest.
5. **Sodium bicarbonate** 1 mEq/kg
   Class IIa
   - If known preexisting bicarbonate response acidosis
   - If overdose with tricyclic antidepressants
   - To alkalinize the urine in drug overdoses
   Class IIb
   - If intubation and continued long arrest interval
   - Upon return of spontaneous circulation after long arrest interval
   Class III
   - Hypoxic lactic acidosis
6. If patient remains in asystole or other agonal rhythm after successful intubation and initial medications and no reversible causes are identified, consider termination of resusitative efforts by a physician. Consider interval since arrest.

Figure 13–5. The asystole algorithm. The critical actions for Case 5: Asystole, are detailed herein. (Algorithm copyright 1992, American Medical Association; JAMA, October 28, 1992; pp 2199–2241.)

CASE 6: ACUTE MYOCARDIAL INFARCTION/THE ACUTE MYOCARDIAL INFARCTION ALGORITHM

Case Setting

Figure 13–6, the acute myocardial infarction algorithm, delineates the ACLS management of patients with signs and symptoms of possible acute MI.

Acute Myocardial Infarction Algorithm
Recommendations for early management of patients with chest pain and possible AMI

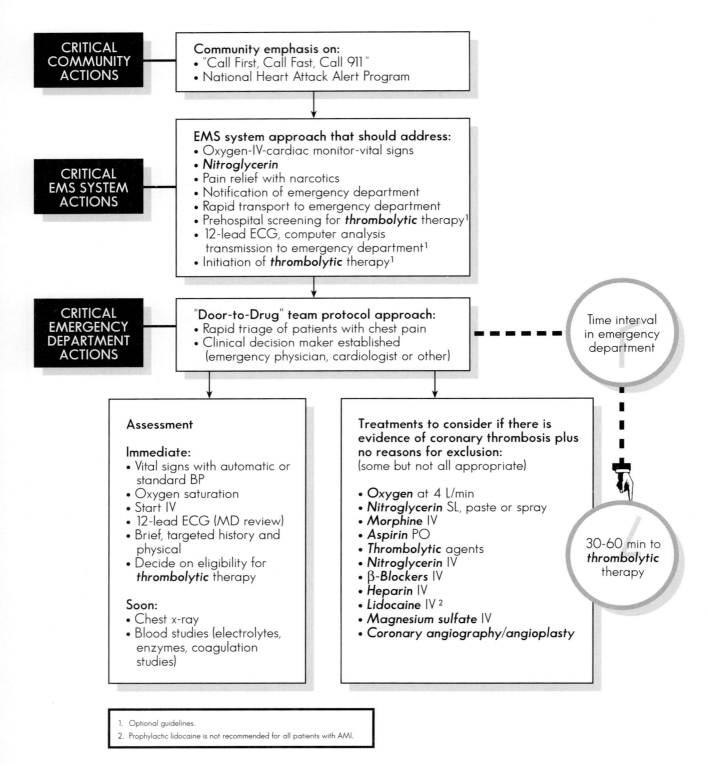

Figure 13–6. The acute myocardial infarction algorithm. The critical actions for Case 6, Acute Myocardial Infarction, are detailed in this algorithm. (Algorithm copyright 1992, American Medical Association; JAMA, October 28, 1992; pp 2199–2241.)

Specific responsibilities of the community at large, the EMS system, and of hospital emergency room staff are highlighted.

Correspondingly, this case is designed to track one "patient" from a pre-hospital setting, such as his or her home, where EMS system responders arrive to provide initial care and transport to the emergency department. In these *three settings*, the victim is evaluated and treated, if so indicated, with a number of agents, including *thrombolytic agents*.

The ACLS instructor can approach this case in any number of ways depending on the background and needs of course participants.

The Scenario

This case develops in stages as the victim encounters the EMS system and is transported to the hospital emergency department for definitive diagnosis and treatment.

ACLS course participants must demonstrate an understanding of the responsibilities of health care providers in the pre-hospital and hospital settings. It is important that course participants demonstrate knowledge of local community standards of care in dealing with suspected AMI victims.

For example, one community may have implemented computer-assisted pre-hospital screening for thrombolytic therapy. In contrast, another may not have paramedic responders administer PO aspirin. Similarly, the "door-to-drug interval" is expected to vary from community to community. It may even vary markedly within the same community.

Critical Performance Skills

What You MUST Do

This case involves hypothetical patients who experience chest pain and other signs and symptoms of AMI in the pre-hospital setting. It is designed to emphasize the importance of early recognition of signs and symptoms and early access to the EMS system.

To demonstrate proficiency at this station, course participants must demonstrate an understanding of the following multipronged approach as outlined in Figure 13–6, the acute myocardial infarction algorithm:

- Know the classic signs and symptoms of possible AMI:
  Chest pain
  Nausea, shortness of breath, and feeling of impending doom
  Gender-related denial
- Know the importance of early access with regard to morbidity and mortality
- Demonstrate an understanding of the following critical EMS system actions:
  Oxygen–IV–cardiac monitor–vital signs
  Nitroglycerin
  Pain relief with narcotics

Notification of emergency department

Rapid transport to emergency department

Pre-hospital screening for thrombolytic therapy

- Know the importance of the "door-to-drug" approach to thrombolytic therapy in the emergency department
- Know the ECG signs of myocardial ischemia, injury, and infarct
- Know the absolute and relative contraindications for thrombolytic therapy
- Know the indications, actions, dosage, and hazards of the following in the setting of possible AMI:

Oxygen

Nitroglycerin SL, paste or spray

Morphine IV

Aspirin PO

Thrombolytic agents

Nitroglycerin IV

Beta blockers IV

Heparin IV

Lidocaine IV

Magnesium sulfate IV

Coronary angioplasty (PCTA)

- Ability to recognize essential ACLS arrhythmias as discussed in Chapters 10, 11, and 12; ability to discuss their treatment in the context of AMI.

What You Must NOT Do

The AHA's *Instructor's Manual for ACLS* considers the following unacceptable performance errors:

- Not recognizing the importance of assessment (ECG, physical examination, history, and vital signs) of the patient with signs and symptoms of possible AMI.
- Not recommending prompt treatment of possible myocardial ischemia with oxygen, nitroglycerin, and morphine.
- Not recommending a 12-lead ECG for determining the extent of myocardial injury and the need for thrombolytic therapy.
- Not determining the presence of absolute and/or relative contraindications to the use of thrombolytic agents.
- Improper or unsafe administration of therapeutic agents or modalities.

CASE 7: UNSTABLE BRADYCARDIA/THE BRADYCARDIA ALGORITHM

Case Setting

Guidelines set forth in the American Heart Association's *Instructor's Manual for Advanced Cardiac Life Support* recommend that Case 7, Unstable Bradycardia, can be placed in one or more of the following settings:

- An unmonitored pre-hospital setting
- An unmonitored emergency department setting
- An unmonitored hospital setting
- A monitored critical care unit setting

Therein, a variety of patient care scenarios can be presented to evaluate the course participants' ability to perform the differential diagnosis of the bradycardias and to correspondingly determine an acceptable therapeutic intervention sequence.

The Scenario

These cases are based on actions outlined in Figure 13–7, the bradycardia algorithm, which is designed to guide the management of symptomatic bradycardias.

The ACLS instructor's manual presents the following case scenario to evaluate course participants' ability to manage these patients.

This scenario, which is typical of a symptomatic bradycardia resulting from AMI, develops as follows:

1. Presenting signs and symptoms:
   Pulse approximately 35 to 40/min
   BP approximately 75/50 mm Hg
   Shortness of breath
   Cold and diaphoretic skin
   Complaint of weakness and light-headedness
2. *Initial ECG:* Second-degree type II AV block with an infranodal block.
3. *Subsequent ECG:* Third-degree AV block.
4. At this point, preparations are begun for a *transvenous pacemaker.*
5. Atropine is initially successful in managing symptoms.
6. *Concurrently,* a TCP is to be placed and capture achieved after proper patient sedation.
7. Also concurrently, a dopamine drip is to be set up on a standby basis should TCP not provide adequate stabilization.

Critical Performance Skills

What You MUST Do

This case presents an opportunity to emphasize major points in managing symptomatic bradycardias. In order to show proficiency at this station, course participants will need to demonstrate the following knowledge and skills:

- Provide oxygen, IV access, and ECG monitoring.
- Assess ECG, BP, and ventilation.
- Determine the presence of symptomatic bradycardia:
   Signs and symptoms must be related to the slow rate
   Symptoms include chest pain, shortness of breath, and altered consciousness

Bradycardia Algorithm
(Patient is not in cardiac arrest)

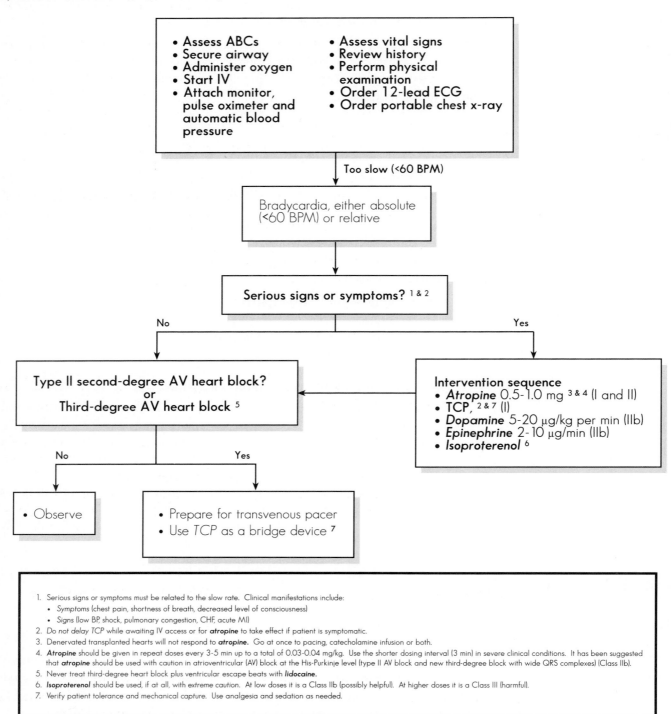

- Assess ABCs
- Secure airway
- Administer oxygen
- Start IV
- Attach monitor, pulse oximeter and automatic blood pressure

- Assess vital signs
- Review history
- Perform physical examination
- Order 12-lead ECG
- Order portable chest x-ray

Too slow (<60 BPM)

Bradycardia, either absolute (<60 BPM) or relative

Serious signs or symptoms? [1 & 2]

No

Yes

Type II second-degree AV heart block?
or
Third-degree AV heart block [5]

Intervention sequence
- *Atropine* 0.5-1.0 mg [3 & 4] (I and II)
- *TCP,* [2 & 7] (I)
- *Dopamine* 5-20 μg/kg per min (IIb)
- *Epinephrine* 2-10 μg/min (IIb)
- *Isoproterenol* [6]

No

Yes

- Observe

- Prepare for transvenous pacer
- Use *TCP* as a bridge device [7]

1. Serious signs or symptoms must be related to the slow rate. Clinical manifestations include:
   - *Symptoms* (chest pain, shortness of breath, decreased level of consciousness)
   - *Signs* (low BP, shock, pulmonary congestion, CHF, acute MI)
2. Do not delay TCP while awaiting IV access or for *atropine* to take effect if patient is symptomatic.
3. Denervated transplanted hearts will not respond to *atropine.* Go at once to pacing, catecholamine infusion or both.
4. *Atropine* should be given in repeat doses every 3-5 min up to a total of 0.03-0.04 mg/kg. Use the shorter dosing interval (3 min) in severe clinical conditions. It has been suggested that *atropine* should be used with caution in atrioventricular (AV) block at the His-Purkinje level (type II AV block and new third-degree block with wide QRS complexes) (Class IIb).
5. Never treat third-degree heart block plus ventricular escape beats with *lidocaine.*
6. *Isoproterenol* should be used, if at all, with *extreme caution.* At low doses it is a Class IIb (possibly helpful). At higher doses it is a Class III (harmful).
7. Verify patient tolerance and mechanical capture. Use analgesia and sedation as needed.

Figure 13–7. The bradycardia algorithm. The critical actions for Case 7, Bradycardia, are detailed in this algorithm. (Algorithm copyright 1992, American Medical Association; JAMA, October 28, 1992; pp 2199–2241.)

Signs include systolic BP less than 80 mm Hg, cold diaphoretic extremities, AMI, and CHF

- Prepare for transvenous pacemaker if *infranodal* second-degree type II or third-degree block exists.
- Stabilize symptomatic bradycardias with atropine initially *while concurrently setting up a TCP.*

  Atropine provides temporary stabilization at best

  Atropine should be used with caution in patients with AV blocks at the infranodal level
- Stabilization with TCP should be achieved as soon as possible, as this modality is a class I intervention for *all* symptomatic bradycardias.

  TCP should not be delayed while awaiting IV access or for atropine to take effect if symptoms exist
- Set up a dopamine drip as a back-up modality should the patient not respond to atropine and should TCP not provide capture or be unavailable.

  The infusion rate for dopamine is 2 to 20 μg/kg/min
- Order a 12-lead ECG to evaluate:

  Extent of myocardial ischemia injury and infarct

  Need for thrombolytic therapy

What You Must NOT Do

The current AHA's *Instructor's Manual for ACLS* cites the following as unacceptable performance errors:

- Administration of atropine or TCP to an asymptomatic bradycardia.
- Not administering atropine while TCP is being established to provide initial stabilization.
- Not recognizing the indications for transvenous pacing.
- Administering isoproterenol instead of dopamine or epinephrine.
- Administering lidocaine to treat ventricular escape beats in third-degree AV block.

CASE 8: UNSTABLE TACHYCARDIA/THE ELECTRICAL CARDIOVERSION ALGORITHM

Case Setting

Guidelines set forth in the American Heart Association's *Instructor's Manual for Advanced Cardiac Life Support* recommend that case studies for evaluating unstable tachycardias be set in one or more of the following settings:

- An unmonitored pre-hospital setting
- An unmonitored emergency department setting
- An unmonitored hospital setting
- A monitored critical care unit setting

Therein, a variety of patient care scenarios can be presented to evaluate course participants' ability to perform the differential diagnosis of unstable tachycardias and to correspondingly determine an acceptable therapeutic intervention sequence.

The Scenario

These cases are based on actions outlined in Figure 13–8, the electrical cardioversion/unstable tachycardia algorithm.

Electrical Cardioversion/Unstable Tachycardia Algorithm
(Patient not in cardiac arrest)

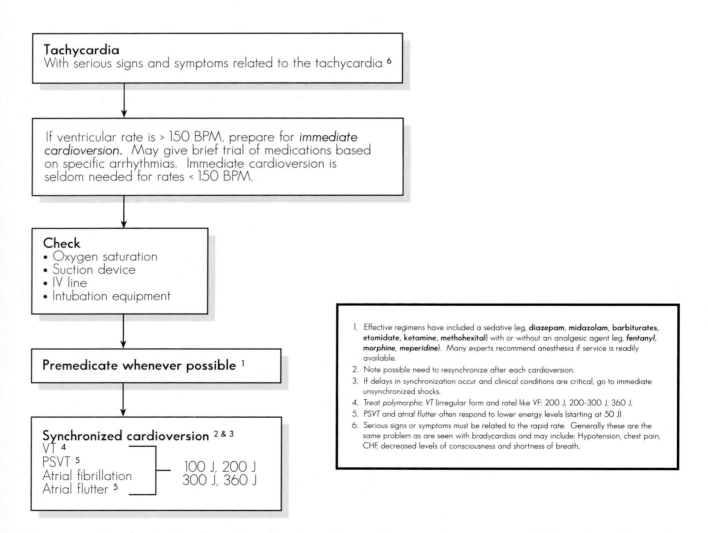

Tachycardia
With serious signs and symptoms related to the tachycardia [6]

If ventricular rate is > 150 BPM, prepare for *immediate cardioversion*. May give brief trial of medications based on specific arrhythmias. Immediate cardioversion is seldom needed for rates < 150 BPM.

Check
• Oxygen saturation
• Suction device
• IV line
• Intubation equipment

Premedicate whenever possible [1]

Synchronized cardioversion [2 & 3]
VT [4]
PSVT [5]
Atrial fibrillation
Atrial flutter [5]   — 100 J, 200 J
                          300 J, 360 J

1. Effective regimens have included a sedative (eg, **diazepam, midazolam, barbiturates, etomidate, ketamine, methohexital**) with or without an analgesic agent (eg, **fentanyl, morphine, meperidine**). Many experts recommend anesthesia if service is readily available.
2. Note possible need to resynchronize after each cardioversion.
3. If delays in synchronization occur and clinical conditions are critical, go to immediate unsynchronized shocks.
4. Treat *polymorphic VT* (irregular form and rate) like VF: 200 J, 200-300 J, 360 J.
5. *PSVT* and *atrial flutter* often respond to lower energy levels (starting at 50 J)
6. Serious signs or symptoms must be related to the rapid rate. Generally these are the same problem as are seen with bradycardias and may include: Hypotension, chest pain, CHF, decreased levels of consciousness and shortness of breath.

Failure 13–8. The electrical cardioversion algorithm. The critical actions for Case 8, Unstable Tachycardia, are detailed in this algorithm. (Algorithm copyright 1992, American Medical Association; JAMA, October 28, 1992; pp 2199–2241.)

The current AHA Instructor's Manual for ACLS recommends cases which evaluate the following unstable tachycardias:

1. *PSVT* (rate of approximately 190/min)
2. *VT* (rate of approximately 170/min)
3. *Torsade de pointes/polymorphic VT* (rate of approximately 170/min)

For all of these cases, the following serious signs and symptoms exist:

1. BP approximately 75/50
2. Complaint of palpitations
3. Cold and diaphoretic extremities
4. Shortness of breath
5. Chest pain
6. Fear and light-headedness

Critical Performance Skills

What You MUST Do

This performance station emphasizes important points in managing patients with unstable tachycardias. In order to demonstrate proficiency, course participants must exhibit the following knowledge and skills:

- Evaluate ABCs, provide oxygen, IV access, and ECG monitoring.
- Assess ECG, BP, and respirations.
- Determine the presence of unstable tachycardia. Remember serious signs and symptoms:
    Must be related to the rapid rate.
    Are *seldom present* at rates less than 150/min.
    Are *not always present* at rates greater than 150/min.
    Include chest pain; dyspnea; altered levels of consciousness; systolic BP less than 80 mm Hg; cold, diaphoretic extremities; and evidence of AMI and/or CHF
- Identify the patient's electrocardiographic rhythm.
- Perform synchronized cardioversion as indicated:
    Observe all proper *safety* and operational procedures
    Synchronize after each shock if necessary
    Use proper energy sequence for each rhythm
- Properly monitor the patient during and after the cardioversion procedure:
    Immediately proceed with defibrillation whenever pulseless VT or VF is detected or should delays in synchronization occur and clinical conditions are critical
    Recognize the need to proceed with or terminate cardioversion efforts based on changes in the patients ECG rhythm
- Properly manage the patient in the postcardioversion phase:
    Assure patient stability by monitoring ABCs, ECG, and vital signs as necessary

Assure patient stability with oxygen, IV fluids, and appropriate antiarrhythmics

What You Must NOT Do

The AHA *Instructor's Manual for ACLS* cites the following as unacceptable performance errors:

- Failure to resynchronize after each shock if necessary
- Failure to immediately defibrillate VF or pulseless VT
- Failure to immediately go to unsynchronized shocks if delays in synchronization occur and clinical conditions are critical
- Failure to identify hemodynamic stability or instability
- Failure to properly identify the patients rhythm
- Treating the monitor, *not* the patient
- Failure to properly manage the patient in the postcardioversion phase

CASE 9: STABLE TACHYCARDIA/THE STABLE TACHYCARDIA ALGORITHM

Case Setting

Guidelines set forth in the American Heart Association's *Instructor's Manual for Advanced Cardiac Life Support* recommend that case studies for evaluating stable tachycardias be set in one or more of the following settings:

- An unmonitored pre-hospital setting
- An unmonitored emergency department setting
- An unmonitored hospital setting
- A monitored critical care unit setting

Therein, a variety of patient care scenario can be presented to evaluate course participants' ability to perform the differential diagnosis of stable tachycardias and to correspondingly determine an acceptable therapeutic intervention sequence.

The Scenario

These cases are based on actions outlined in Figure 13–9, the stable tachycardia algorithm.

The current AHA's *Instructor's Manual for ACLS* recommends cases which evaluate the following stable tachycardias:

1. *PSVT* with a rate of 160/min
2. *Wide-complex tachycardia* of uncertain origin with a rate of 160/min
3. *VT* with a rate of 160/min
4. *Atrial flutter/atrial fibrillation* with a rate of 160/min

Tachycardia Algorithm

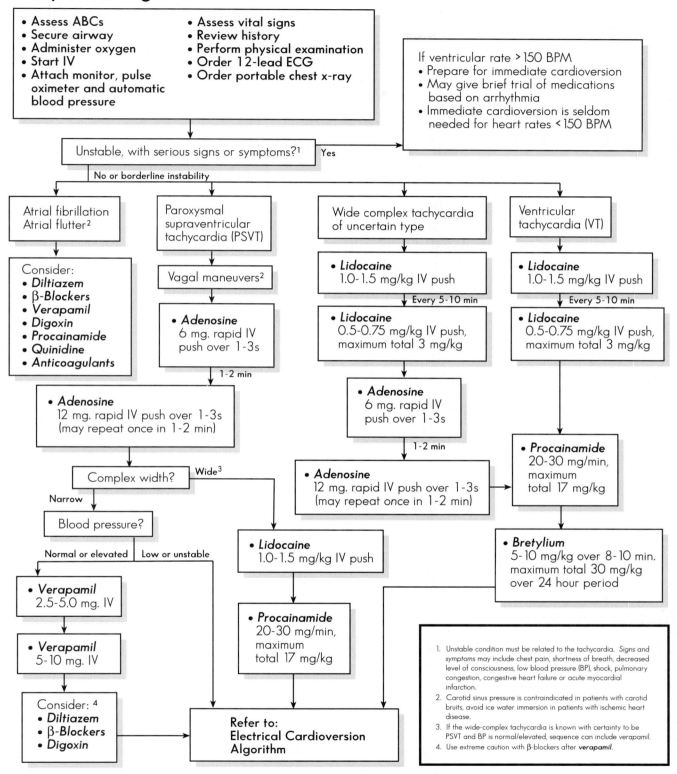

Figure 13–9. The stable tachycardia algorithm. The critical actions for Case 9: Stable Tachycardia, are detailed in this algorithm. (Algorithm copyright 1992, American Medical Association; JAMA, October 28, 1992; pp 2199–2241.)

For these cases, hemodynamic stability is evidenced by the presence of the following clinical signs and symptoms:

1. BP in the range of 120/80
2. No complaint of chest pain or shortness of breath
3. Alertness and orientation
4. Clear lungs on auscultation
5. No *cartoid bruits*

Critical Performance Skills

What You MUST Do

This performance station emphasizes important points in managing the patient with a stable tachycardia. In order to demonstrate proficiency, course participants must exhibit the following knowledge and skills:

- Evaluate ABCs, provide oxygen, IV access, and ECG monitoring.
- Assess ECG, BP, and respiration.
- Determine hemodynamic stability or instability.
    Serious signs and symptoms are *seldom* present at heart rates less than 150/min.
    If the heart rate is greater than 150/min and the patient is hemodynamically stable, *treat the patient, not the monitor.*
- Identify the patient's ECG rhythm.
- Perform correctly the intervention sequence for each of the following rhythms as directed by the stable tachycardia algorithm (Figure 13–9):
    PSVT
    VT
    Wide-complex tachycardias of uncertain origin
    Atrial flutter/atrial fibrillation
- Demonstrate the ability to properly cardiovert the above rhythm if so indicated.
- Continue to monitor ABCs and vital signs as rhythm changes are noted in response to therapeutic interventions.

What You Must NOT Do

The AHA's *Instructor's Manual for ACLS* cites the following as unacceptable errors:

- Failure to properly determine the presence or absence of hemodynamic stability
- Failure to properly identify the patient's rhythm
- Failure to employ correct intervention sequence as outlined in Figure 13–9
- Failure to listen for cartoid bruits prior to performing cartoid massage
- Treating the monitor, *not* the patient

BIBLIOGRAPHY

1. American Heart Association. Emergency Cardiac Care Committee and Subcommittees. Guidelines for cardiopulmonary resuscitation and emergency cardiac care. JAMA 1992;268:2171–2295
2. American Heart Association. Textbook of advanced cardiac life support. Dallas, TX: American Heart Association, 1994
3. American Heart Association. Instructor's manual for advanced cardiac life support. Dallas, TX: American Heart Association, 1994
4. Billi JE. The educational direction of the ACLS training program. Ann Emerg Med 1993;22(Part 2):484–488
5. Billi JE, Membrino GE, Education in ACLS training programs: changing the paradigm. Ann Emerg Med 1993;22(Part 2):475–483

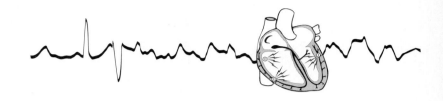

ESSENTIALS OF ACLS
POST-TEST

1. What percentage of deaths from myocardial infarction occur before the patient reaches the hospital?
   a. 10
   b. 33
   c. 25
   d. over 50

2. Although responses vary, in general, moderate doses (5 to 10 μg/kg/min) of dopamine result in
   a. renal arteriolar vasodilatation
   b. increases in cardiac output
   c. tachycardia
   d. marked increases in systemic vascular resistance

3. Verapamil may be harmful in the treatment of
   a. ventricular tachycardia (VT)
   b. atrial flutter
   c. atrial fibrillation
   d. PSVT

4. Useful drugs for the emergency treatment of cardiogenic shock include
   1. norepinephrine
   2. morphine
   3. dopamine
   4. furosemide
   a. 1, 3, 4
   b. 2, 3, 4

c. 1, 2, 3
d. 1, 3

5. Which of the following agents have a favorable effect on the fibrillatory threshold?
   1. lidocaine
   2. procainamide
   3. oxygen
   4. atropine
   a. 1, 3
   b. 2, 3, 4
   c. 1, 2, 3
   d. all of the above

6. Which of the following modalities or agents may enhance electrical conversion in the presence of refractory ventricular fibrillation?
   1. oxygen
   2. hyperventilation
   3. morphine
   4. epinephrine
   a. 1, 2, 3
   b. 1, 3, 4
   c. 1, 2, 4
   d. all of the above

7. Nitroglycerin has which of the following actions?
   1. reduces left ventricular afterload
   2. decreases venous return
   3. increases ventricular inotropicity
   4. improves coronary arterial blood flow
   a. 1, 2, 3
   b. 1, 3
   c. 1, 2, 4
   d. all of the above

8. Epinephrine
   1. increases aortic blood pressure
   2. can restore spontaneous contractions in asystole
   3. widens the fibrillatory threshold
   4. enhances defibrillation in ventricular fibrillation
   a. 1, 2, 4
   b. 1, 2, 3
   c. 1, 3, 4
   d. all of the above

9. The airway of choice for an unconscious patient with adequate spontaneous ventilations is an
   a. oropharyngeal airway
   b. nasopharyngeal airway
   c. endotracheal tube
   d. esophageal airway

10. Ways of minimizing the hazards of endotracheal intubation during cardiac arrest include
    1. not using the teeth as a fulcrum
    2. limiting attempts to 30 seconds
    3. hyperventilating and hyperoxygenating between attempts
    4. application of cricoid pressure
    a. 1, 2, 3
    b. 3, 4
    c. 1, 2, 4
    d. all of the above

11. Which of the following are true statements regarding curved and straight laryngoscope blades?
    1. the straight blade is designed to lift the epiglottis
    2. the curved blade allows visualization of the vocal cords without displacing the epiglottis
    3. the straight blade is used primarily for placement of nasogastric tubes
    4. both blades contain small lamps which may pose an aspiration danger
    a. 1, 3
    b. 2, 4
    c. 1, 4
    d. 2, 3

12. Which of the following best describe the ideal position of the patient for endotracheal intubation?
    a. patient supine, head elevated with flexion of neck and extension of head
    b. patient supine, head flexed and neck extended
    c. patient supine, head elevated with hyperextension of the neck
    d. patient supine, with head and neck flexed

13. Advantages of endotracheal intubation during ACLS include
    1. reduces risk of gastric aspiration
    2. allows administration of 100% oxygen
    3. provides an effective route of administration for selected drugs
    4. allows hyperventilation and management of acidosis
    a. 1, 2, 3
    b. 2, 3, 4
    c. 1, 3, 4
    d. all of the above

14. Hazards of endotracheal intubation include
    1. endobronchial intubation
    2. esophageal intubation
    3. damage to teeth
    4. hypoxia during procedure
    a. 1, 2, 4
    b. 1, 3, 4
    c. 2, 3, 4
    d. all of the above

15. The nasopharyngeal airway is
    a. better tolerated in semicomatose patients than the oropharyngeal
       airway
    b. inserted upside down, and then rotated 360°
    c. used to push the tongue posteriorly
    d. designed for use in patients with coagulopathies

16. Select the incorrect statement regarding self-inflating bag–valve–mask
    adult manual resuscitation units.
    a. oxygen flow rates are generally set at 12 to 15 L/min
    b. an oxygen reservoir is used to improve oxygen delivery
    c. clear masks are recommended
    d. 50-cm H_2O pop-off devices are required

17. Present evidence indicates that the dose of epinephrine injected in the
    tracheobronchial tree should be
    a. 0.25 mg diluted with 10 mL of solution
    b. 0.5 mg diluted with 10 mL of solution
    c. 1.0 mg diluted with 10 mL of solution
    d. 2.0 mg diluted with 10 mL of solution

18. Lidocaine
    1. may not be administered endotracheally
    2. widens the fibrillatory threshold
    3. is indicated in unstable VT
    4. is not part of the routine management of AMI
    a. 1, 4
    b. 2, 3
    c. 1, 3
    d. 2, 4

19. In the management of stable VT, which of the following is the correct sequence for lidocaine?
    a. 1.0 to 1.5 mg/kg followed by half the initial dose up to a maximum dose of 3.0 mg/kg
    b. 0.5 to 1.0 mg/kg followed by half the initial dose up to a maximum dose of 3.0 mg/kg
    c. 1.0 to 1.5 mg/kg; this dose may be repeated up to a maximum of 3.0 mg/kg
    d. 0.5 to 1.0 mg/kg followed by half the initial dose up to a maximum of 30 to 35 mg/kg

20. When administered in a continuous infusion following successful defibrillation, the correct dosage for lidocaine is
    a. 1 to 2 mg/min
    b. 2 to 4 mg/min
    c. 2 to 4 mg/kg/min
    d. 1 to 2 mg/kg/min

21. Common adverse reactions to adenosine include
    1. hypotension
    2. chest pain
    3. flushing
    4. speeding of ventricular rate
    a. 1, 2, 3
    b. 2, 3, 4
    c. 1, 2, 4
    d. all of the above

22. A 45-year-old patient is brought to the emergency department with a complaint of palpitations. The BP is 110/70 mm Hg and the monitor shows PSVT with a rate of 190/min. The next course of action is to
    a. perform cartoid sinus massage
    b. administer adenosine
    c. auscultate for carotid bruits
    d. administer verapamil

23. While preparing for synchronized cardioversion, the monitor reveals ventricular fibrillation. The patient is oriented to person and place. Your response is to
    a. perform synchronized countershocks immediately
    b. confirm the rhythm in more than one lead
    c. defibrillate immediately
    d. begin CPR

24. An 80-kg patient is brought to the emergency department with complaints of nausea and vertigo. After 1.0 mg of atropine, the ECG shows sinus bradycardia with a rate of 45/min and the BP is 85/60 mm Hg. Your next course of action would be to administer
    a. dopamine 5 to 20 μg/kg/min
    b. epinephrine 2 to 10 μg/kg
    c. isoproterenol 2 to 10 μg/kg
    d. atropine 0.5 to 1.0 mg IV bolus

25. Magnesium sulfate
    1. is a treatment of choice for Torsade de pointes
    2. 1 to 2 g IV given over 1 to 2 min may be indicated in refractory VF/VT
    3. hypertension is a frequently noted side effect
    4. 1 to 2 g IV given over 5 to 60 min may be indicated post-MI
    a. 1, 2, 4
    b. 1, 2, 3
    c. 2, 3, 4
    d. all of the above

26. True statements regarding IV techniques during ACLS include
    1. administration of drugs should be followed by a fluid bolus and elevation of the extremity
    2. a volume infusion is not a routine part of the treatment of cardiac arrest
    3. 5% dextrose is the preferred infusion solution during cardiac arrest
    4. intracardiac drug administration is not advised during ACLS
    a. 1, 3, 4
    b. 1, 2, 4
    c. 2, 3, 4
    d. all of the above

27. Potentially adverse outcomes related to transcutaneous pacing (TCP) include
    1. patient discomfort
    2. pacer-induced artifact obscuring dangerous rhythms
    3. delays in achieving capture
    4. erythema
    a. 1, 2, 4
    b. 1, 2, 3
    c. 2, 3, 4
    d. all of the above

28. A 35-year-old patient with a complaint of palpitations is seen in the emergency department. The BP is 120/80, and the monitor shows a narrow complex PSVT with a rate of 180/min. The patient has not responded to vagal maneuvers or a 6-mg IV dose of adenosine. The next intervention would be
    a. adenosine 12 mg rapid IV push
    b. verapamil 2.5 to 5 mg IV
    c. synchronized cardioversion at 100 J
    d. lidocaine 1.0 to 1.5 mg/kg IV push

29. A patient with a complaint of chest pain is brought to the emergency department. Oxygen, sublingual nitroglycerin, and morphine IV, are given. The BP is 100/60 mm Hg, and the monitor shows ventricular bi and trigemine. Your intervention would be
    a. synchronized cardioversion
    b. lidocaine 1 to 2 mg/min continuous infusion
    c. lidocaine 1 to 1.5 mg/kg IV push
    d. procainamide 30 mg/min IV infusion

30. Select the *incorrect* dosing schedule for treatment of refractory VF/VT.
    a. lidocaine 1.0 to 1.5 mg/kg. Repeat in 3 to 5 min to total dose of 3 mg/kg
    b. procainamide 30 mg/min to a maximum total of 17 mg/kg
    c. bretylium 5 mg/kg; repeat in 5 min at 10 mg/kg to a maximum dose of 30 to 35 mg/kg
    d. magnesium sulfate 1 to 2 g over 5 to 60 min

31. Select the *incorrect* dosing schedule for stable VT.
    a. lidocaine 1 to 1.5 mg; repeat in 5 to 10 min at 1 to 1.5 mg/kg to a maximum total dose of 3 mg/kg
    b. procainamide 20 to 30 mg/min to a maximum total of 17 mg/kg
    c. bretylium 5 to 10 mg/kg over 8 to 10 min to a maximum total of 30 mg over 24 hr
    d. synchronized cardioversion at 100 J, 200 J, 300 J, 360 J

32. Beta-blocking agents would be *least* advisable during which of the following situations?
    a. acute cardiogenic shock
    b. atrial fibrillation
    c. postmyocardial infarction
    d. atrial flutter

33. Which of the following is considered *least* useful for treating myocardial ischemia due to possible AMI?
    a. oxygen
    b. lidocaine
    c. morphine
    d. nitroglycerin

34. Which of the following agents may be employed to reduce thrombus size or reformation?
    1. streptokinase IV
    2. aspirin PO
    3. beta blockers
    4. heparin IV
    a. 1, 3, 4
    b. 1, 2, 4
    c. 1, 2, 3
    d. all of the above

35. In order not to interfere with an automated external defibrillator's rhythm analysis process, efforts should be made to minimize or eliminate which of the following sources of signal artifact?
    1. respiratory efforts
    2. gross patient movement
    3. transport vehicle movement
    4. CPR
    a. 2, 3, 4
    b. 1, 3, 4
    c. 1, 2, 3
    d. all of the above

36. Which of the following is the *least* treatable cause of pulseless electrical activity (PEA)?
    a. hypovolemia
    b. cardiac tamponade
    c. massive pulmonary embolism
    d. tension pneumothorax

37. Stable atrial fibrillation would best be treated with which one of the following agents?
    a. dobutamine
    b. diltiazem
    c. atropine
    d. lidocaine

38. Signs that PEA may be due to tension pneumothorax include
    1. flat neck veins
    2. weak or absent pulse during CPR
    3. unilateral breath sounds and/or tracheal deviation
    4. florid face
    a. 1, 2, 4
    b. 2, 3, 4
    c. 2, 4
    d. all of the above

39. Post successful resuscitation from VF/VT, which of the following would be *least* advisable?
    a. oxygen
    b. lidocaine 1.0 mg/kg IV as a loading dose
    c. lidocaine continuous infusion at 2 to 4 mg/min
    d. epinephrine 2 to 10 mg/min infusion

40. A patient with wide-complex third-degree AV block is seen in the emergency department. The BP is 70/40 mm Hg. The ventricular rate is 30/min. Which of the following is the *definitive* intervention?
    a. atropine
    b. transcutaneous pacemaker (TCP)
    c. transvenous pacemaker (TVP)
    d. dopamine infusion

41. A patient with PEA is intubated and being ventilated at a rate of 15/min. With compressions stopped, an end-tidal CO_2 monitor reads 20 mm Hg. This would indicate
    a. esophageal intubation
    b. some perfusion exists
    c. compressions be resumed
    d. absence of perfusion

42. Select the *false* statement regarding endotracheal suctioning.
    a. hypoxemia may trigger tachycardia
    b. bradyarrhythmias can be caused by vagal stimulation
    c. pulse rate is monitored
    d. vacuum is set between 40 and 180 mm Hg

43. Complications specific to the use of catheter-through-needle devices include
    a. interruption of CPR
    b. infection
    c. hematoma formation
    d. catheter fragment embolism

44. A patient with PEA is seen in ICU. The monitor reveals a sinus rhythm with a rate of 90/min. Which of the following interventions is least advisable?
    a. volume infusion
    b. intubation
    c. checking of breath sounds
    d. atropine 0.5 to 1.0 mg IV bolus

45. Dobutamine infusion at 10 µg/kg/min
    1. increases cardiac output
    2. increases myocardial contractility
    3. increases blood pressure via increased peripheral resistance
    4. may increase myocardial oxygen requirement
    a. 1, 4
    b. 1, 2, 4
    c. 1, 2, 3
    d. all of the above

46. Adverse reactions to lidocaine IV include
    1. altered consciousness
    2. muscle tremors and seizures
    3. VT
    4. slowing of conduction through the AV node
    a. 1, 2
    b. 3, 4
    c. 1, 4
    d. 2, 3

47. A patient is seen in the emergency department following an automobile accident. Multiple traumas exist including rib fractures and facial, head, and neck injuries. In addition, active bleeding is noted from several large lacerations. Your immediate priority is to
    a. achieve hemostasis
    b. provide chest wall stability
    c. open the airway
    d. check for pulselessness

48. Torsade de pointes may result from overadministration of which of the following ACLS drugs?
    1. procainamide
    2. digitalis
    3. quinidine
    4. magnesium sulfate
    a. 1, 3
    b. 2, 3
    c. 1, 4
    d. 2, 4

49. A patient with PEA is seen in the emergency department. He has jugular venous distention, and no pulse can be felt during CPR. Breath sounds are equal while being ventilated with 100% oxygen. After two 250-mL fluid challenges, the BP, assessed by Doppler device at the femoral vein, is 60/p. You would recommend
    a. emergency pericardiocentesis
    b. an echocardiogram
    c. needle decompression
    d. 100-mL volume infusion

50. A patient is seen in the emergency department with a wide-complex tachycardia of uncertain origin. After two doses of lidocaine and two additional doses of adenosine, the patient's heart rate is 220/min and the BP is 70/40 mm Hg. At this point, the patient shows signs of marked CNS depression. You would now recommend
    a. procainamide 20 to 30 mg/min
    b. bretylium 5 to 10 mg/kg over 8 to 10 min
    c. synchronized cardioversion at 50 to 100 J
    d. synchronized cardioversion at 200 J

ESSENTIALS OF ACLS POST-TEST: WRITTEN REFERENCED ANSWERS

The questions presented in the foregoing test were constructed to measure the same knowledge and skills as do the items on the actual ACLS written examination.

To help course participants prepare for the ACLS examination process, each question is discussed and referenced to the following AHA publications.

Reference I: American Heart Association. Guidelines for CPR and ECC. JAMA 1992;268:2171–2302

Reference II: American Heart Association. Textbook for advanced cardiac life support. Dallas, TX: American Heart Association, 1994

Reference III: American Heart Association. Instructor's manual for ACLS. Dallas, TX: American Heart Association, 1994

Following each discussion, the question will be referenced to one of the three standard texts mentioned above. Following the reference citation (eg, reference I, reference II, etc.) will come the pages(s) or chapter and page number(s) that can be used to obtain additional information.

1. Answer . . . d.

Of the half million or so annual deaths from cardiac arrest in the United States, approximately 300,000 will die before they reach the hospital.

Ref I: page 2174

2. Answer . . . b.

"Cardiac" doses of dopamine (5 to 10 µg/kg/min) usually produce increased cardiac output without increasing systemic vascular resistance. At "renal" doses (2 to 5 µ/kg/min) the result is renal arteriolar dilatation. "Vasopressor" doses (greater than 10 mg/kg/min) cause SVR to increase and can produce unwanted tachycardia.

Ref I: page 2209

3. Answer . . . a.

The administration of verapamil to a patient with VT can be a lethal error. This agent is useful in the management of stable narrow-complex supraventricular tachycardias.

Ref I: pages 2222–2224

4. Answer . . . d.

As morphine and furosemide can cause systemic vascular resistance to drop, their use is not advisable in the management of cardiogenic shock.

Ref I: pages 2226–2228

5. Answer . . . c.

Atropine's positive chronotropic action will increase myocardial oxygen demand. Lidocaine and procainamide slow the rate of automaticity of ectopic pacemaker cells. Oxygen is the classic anti-ischemic agent.

Ref I: pages 2205–2208

6. Answer . . . c.

When VF/VT is refractory to three initial attempts at defibrillation, considerable pathology is felt to exist. Hyperventilation with 100% oxygen can help manage acidosis. Epinephrine is felt to facilitate the myocardial response to unsynchronized countershock.

Ref I: pages 2215–2219

7. Answer . . . c.

Nitroglycerin, by producing arteriolar and venular vasodilatation reduces both left heart pre- and afterload. These beneficial effects are felt to reduce ischemia and infarct size.

Ref I: page 2210

8. Answer . . . a.

Most of the beneficial actions of epinephrine in cardiac arrest are due to its alpha-adrenergic action which increases mean aortic pressure and, hence, cerebral and coronary blood flow. Its use can increase myocardial oxygen consumption and thus narrow the fibrillatory threshold.

Ref I: page 2208

9. Answer . . . a.

Oropharyngeal airways cannot be used on semiconscious patients as they can stimulate vomiting. Adequate spontaneous ventilations preclude endotracheal intubation.

Ref I: pages 2199–2203

10. Answer . . . d.

All of the actions indicated in this question are vital to minimizing complications of the intubation procedure in the setting of ACLS.

Ref II: Chapter 2, pages 3–6

11. Answer . . . c.

Visualization of the vocal cords necessitates anterior displacement of the epiglottis. The straight blade is placed under it and thus *lifts* it out of the way. The curved blade is placed in the vallecula allowing anterior displacement.

Ref II: Chapter 2, pages 3–6

12. Answer . . . a.

The patient is placed in the "sniffing" position. The head is first elevated with a folded towel. The neck is then flexed and the head extended. These actions help align the axis of the pharynx, the larynx, and the trachea.

Ref II: Chapter 2, pages 3–6

13. Answer . . . d.

All of the factors mentioned in this question are advantages of endotracheal intubation as a means of securing the airway during ACLS.

Ref II: Chapter 2, pages 3–6

14. Answer . . . d.

All of the problems listed are hazards that can be caused or encountered in providing endotracheal intubation during ACLS.

Ref II: Chapter 2, pages 3–6

15. Answer . . . a.

An advantage of nasopharyngeal airways is that they can be used in conscious and semiconscious patients.

Ref I: page 2201

16. Answer . . . d.

Adult manual rescusitation devices are designed without pop-off valves. This allows them to deliver ventilations through an ET tube that are not synchronized with compressions.

Ref I: page 2200

17. Answer . . . d.

Medications should be given at 2 to 2.5 times the recommended IV dose and should be diluted in 10 mL of normal saline or distilled water.

Ref I: page 2205

18. Answer . . . d.

Given IV or via ET tube, lidocaine suppresses ectopy by widening the fibrillatory threshold. Not part of the routine management of uncomplicated AMI, it should neither be used when VT exists with serious signs and symptoms.

Ref I: page 2206

19. Answer . . . a.

The stable tachycardia algorithm illustrates the sequence outlined in choice a.

Ref I: page 2223

20. Answer . . . b.

For most patients requiring a continuous infusion of lidocaine, a rate of 2 to 4 mg/min is recommended. As with all agents, patients should be observed for toxic effects.

Ref I: page 2206

21. Answer . . . a.

Because its half-life is only 5 seconds, wanted and unwanted actions of adenosine are short lived. This increases its margin of safety in ACLS. Because it slows conduction through the AV node, *slowing* of the ventricular rate must be watched for.

Ref I: page 2207

22. Answer . . . c.

Cartoid sinus pressure is contraindicated in patients with cartoid bruits. Therefore, prior to performing this procedure, the patient's neck vessels must be auscultated for signs of cartoid artery disease.

Ref I: page 2223–2224

23. Answer . . . b.

A patient who is oriented to person and place has a perfusing rhythm! ACLS providers must remember that VF/VT can be mimicked by electrocardiographic artifact. The first and last rule of ACLS is to "treat the patient, not the monitor."

Ref I: pages 2215–2216

24. Answer . . . d.

The dosage end point for atropine is 0.04 mg/kg, which is slightly more than 3.5 mg for an 80-kg patient. Atropine must be given cautiously to patients with myocardial ischemia. Thus, a 12-lead ECG should be performed. Remember, a TCP is always indicated in symptomatic bradycardias; however, achieving capture and patient comfort takes skill.

Ref I: pages 2221–2222

25. Answer . . . a.

When low serum magnesium levels are known or suspected, the abnormality must be corrected, as it can lead to refractory VF/VT, ectopy, and Torsade de pointes. When these conditions exist, 1 to 2 g may be administered over 1 to 2 min.

Ref I: page 2208

26. Answer . . . b.

Normal saline or Ringer's lactate are preferred for infusion during cardiac arrest, although dextrose solutions are acceptable. Fluid challenge can be both diagnostic and therapeutic during PEA but is not part of the routine management of VF/VT or asystole. Intracardiac injections are strongly discouraged during ACLS.

Ref I: page 2205

27. Answer . . . d.

When TCP is indicated, achieving patient comfort and capture requires skill. Skin burns are not uncommon. In older models without electronic filtering circuitry, pacer spike artifact could mask dangerous rhythms.

Ref II: Chapter 5, pages 5–6

28. Answer . . . a.

According to the stable tachycardia algorithm, a second dose of adenosine is indicated when these conditions exist.

Ref I: page 2223

29. Answer . . . c.

This is an example of symptomatic PVCs. They are felt to exist when ectopy does not respond to anti-ischemia measures and probability is good that it is *contributing* to ischemia. In this context, lidocaine (1.0 to 1.5 mg/kg) is indicated.

Ref II: Chapter 1, pages 54–58

30. Answer . . . d.

The correct dosing schedule for magnesium sulfate in refractory VF/VT is 1 to 2 g given over 1 to 2 min.

Ref I: page 2217

31. Answer . . . a

According to the stable tachycardia algorithm, the second dose of lidocaine should be *half* the initial dose or 0.5 to 0.75 mg/kg.

Ref I: page 2223

32. Answer . . . a.

Beta-blocking agents and calcium channel blockers depress the pumping action of the heart and would not be indicated in cardiogenic shock.

Ref I: pages 2226–2229

33. Answer . . . b.

Lidocaine will not treat ischemia. Indeed, it will suppress the ventricular ectopy that often serves as a warning signal that ischemia exists.

Ref II: Chapter 1, pages 54, 58

34. Answer . . . b.

Aspirin, thrombolytic agents, and heparin are all part of the "thrombolytic package" given to patients post-AMI. Aspirin PO helps prevent thrombi from growing. Thrombolytic agents dissolve these clots. Heparin prevents clots from reforming on the injured coronary endothelial cell walls. Beta-blocking agents are used to limit infarct size.

Ref II: Chapter 1, pages 51–53

35. Answer . . . a.

The electronic circuitry on automated external defibrillator (AED) devices can filter out patient respiratory, and much patient movement artifact while in the "analysis" mode. This is not the case with transport vehicle artifact or that due to CPR. Concerted efforts should be made to ensure that movement be minimized during analysis.

Ref II: Chapter 4, page 9

36. Answer . . . c.

Hypovolemia is easily treated. Cardiac tamponade and tension pneumothorax require needle pericardiocentesis and needle decompression respectively. Massive pulmonary embolism requires surgical embolectomy.

Ref I: pages 2219–2220

37. Answer . . . b.

Atrial fibrillation is treated with drugs that slow conduction through the AV node. This helps control the ventricular rate. Calcium channel blockers, beta-blocking agents, and sometimes digitalis are used for rate control.

Ref I: page 2224

38. Answer . . . d.

All of these choices are signs that suggest the presence of tension pneumothorax. Other clues include a history of chest trauma, status asthmaticus, chronic obstructive pulmonary disease (COPD), the presence of central venous lines, and recent CPR.

Ref III: Chapter 9, pages 4–6, 4–7

39. Answer . . . d.

Following resuscitation from VF/VT, lidocaine and oxygen are indicated. Epinephrine is not indicated. This agent increases myocardial oxygen demands. A loading dose of lidocaine followed by a continuous infusion is indicated.

Ref I: page 2206

40. Answer . . . c.

Transvenous pacing is indicated and is the definitive treatment for wide-complex third-degree AV block. These rhythms will usually deteriorate to asystole unless electrical capture can be achieved.

Ref II: Chapter 5, pages 3–4

41. Answer . . . b.

Even with proper tracheal intubation and ventilation, should perfusion not exist, carbon dioxide cannot be eliminated. The use of these devices to detect blood flow in PEA is growing. Blood flow in PEA means that *pseudo-EMD* is present and that chances for survival are enhanced.

Ref I: pages 2202, 2219–2220

42. Answer . . . d.

The suction pressure should be set at between -80 and -120 mm Hg for the adult.

Ref II: Chapter 2, page 15

43. Answer . . . d.

Should the catheter be retracted through these devices, the tip can be sheared off. The result would be a catheter fragment embolism.

Ref II: Chapter 6, page 2

44. Answer . . . d.

Atropine is not indicated in the management of PEA unless the cardiac rate is less than 60/min. The other interventions are part of the nonspecific problem-solving management of PEAs.

Ref I: pages 2219–2220

45. Answer . . . b.

Dobutamine is a potent inotrope without vasopressor activity. Thus, increases in BP seen are *not* due to increases in systemic vascular resistance (SVR). Tachycardias and increased myocardial oxygen demand are often noted at higher doses.

Ref I: page 2209

46. Answer . . . a.

Toxic reactions to lidocaine include slurred speech, altered consciousness, muscle twitching, and seizures. It will treat, not cause, VT and has no effect on conduction through the AV node.

Ref I: page 2206

47. Answer . . . c.

The ACLS provider must never forget the primary and secondary ABCD surveys. The time to analyze an overwhelming or traumatic experience is in a post-code debriefing session. Bleeding is a sign that a perfusing rhythm exists.

Ref II: Chapter 1, pages 5–10

48. Answer . . . a.

Antiarrhythmic drugs, which prolong repolarization and the QT interval, are among the most common causes of torsade. It is also commonly associated with hypomagnesemia, which is why magnesium sulfate is part of its treatment when patient stability and time permit.

Ref II: Chapter 3, page 7

49. Answer . . . a.

The patient's clinical state is critical. The response to a 500-mL volume infusion is typical of cardiac tamponade. Also suggestive of this disorder is JVD and the absence of pulse in response to CPR. Bilateral breath sounds help rule out tension pneumothorax. Time and the immediate threat to life rule out an echocardiogram.

Finally, an additional 100-mL volume infusion is not the response warranted by a life-threatening situation such as this.

Ref III: Chapter 9, pages 4–5, 4–6

50. Answer . . . c.

An unstable VT is indicated by the low BP, the altered consciousness, and the failure to respond to an appropriate intervention sequence. Synchronized cardioversion is indicated.

Ref I: pages 2223–2225

Index